Essentials of Aggression Management in Health Care

WITHDRAWN

Steven S. Wilder, CHSP, EMT-P

Chris Sorensen, CHPA

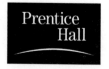

Prentice Hall

Prentice Hall, Upper Saddle River, New Jersey 07458

Library of Congress Cataloging-in-Publication Data
The essentials of aggression management in health care / Steve S. Wilder, Chris Sorensen.
    p. cm.
  Includes index.
  ISBN 0-13-013130-X (alk. paper)
   1. Medical personnel—Crimes against—Prevention. 2. Medical personnel—Safety
measures. 3. Violence in the workplace—Prevention. 4. Aggressiveness. 5. Aggressive
behavior (Psychology)—Prevention. I. Wilder, Steven S. (Steven Scott), 1958- II.
Sorensen, Chris, CHPA

R727.2 .E875 2001
362.1'068—dc21
                                           00-046523

Publisher: Julie Alexander
Executive Editor: Greg Vis
Acquisitions Editor: Katrin Beacom
Production Liaison: Janet Bolton
Production Editor: Barbara J. Barg,
  Navta Associates, Inc.
**Director of Manufacturing
  and Production:** Bruce Johnson
Managing Editor: Patrick Walsh
Manufacturing Manager: Ilene Sanford
Art Director: Marianne Frasco
Marketing Manager: Tiffany Price
Cover Design: Bruce Kenselaar
Cover Coordination: Maria Guglielmo
Photography: Ryland Gagnon,
  Precision Video and Photography, Bradley, IL
Line Art: Chris Capuzzi, Obsession Tattoos
Composition: Navta Associates, Inc.
Printing and Binding: Banta Harrisonburg

Notice: The authors and the publisher of this book have taken care to make certain that the procedures described in this textbook reflect currently accepted practice; however, they cannot be considered absolute recommendations.

It is the reader's responsibility to stay informed of any policy or procedural changes or recommendations made by federal, state, and local agencies, as well as by his or her employing institution or agency. The authors and publisher of this textbook disclaim any liability, loss, injury, damage, or risk resulting directly or indirectly from suggested procedures and theory or any undetected errors in the text, or from readers' misunderstanding of the text. The authors and publisher disclaim any liability, loss, injury, damage, or risk incurred as a consequence, directly or indirectly, from the use and application of any of the contents of this book.

Prentice-Hall International (UK) Limited, *London*
Prentice-Hall of Australia Pty. Limited, *Sydney*
Prentice-Hall Canada Inc., *Toronto*
Prentice-Hall Hispanoamericana, S.A., *Mexico*
Prentice-Hall of India Private Limited, *New Delhi*
Prentice-Hall of Japan, Inc., *Tokyo*
Prentice-Hall Singapore Pte. Ltd.
Editora Prentice-Hall do Brasil, Ltda., *Rio de Janeiro*

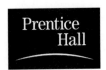

10 9 8 7 6 5 4 3 2 1
ISBN 0-13-013130-X

Essentials of Aggression Management in Health Care

Thanks to our friends and families, for their ongoing support and encouragement.

Contents

9 Types and Uses of Restraints 123

10 Postincident Responses 139

Preface

A nurse in an emergency room is attacked by an enraged patient. A social worker visiting a patient's home in a dangerous neighborhood is attacked by a group of thugs looking for drugs or money. The driver of a vehicle involved in a motor vehicle accident suddenly becomes violent with the paramedic who is treating him. A psychiatric patient corners a nurse and nearly is able to attack her before help arrives. A hospital security officer is stabbed in the abdomen while trying to prevent a group of gang members from entering a treatment area where a fellow gang member is being treated.

Do these incidents sound as if they may have come right from the script of a prime-time television show? Unfortunately, that isn't the case. These are real incidents involving real healthcare providers who found themselves becoming the victims of violent behavior at the hands of patients, visitors, friends, or family members.

Healthcare professionals realize that providing care to the sick and injured has become a dangerous business. More and more providers are finding themselves victims of aggressive behavior. Fire departments, ambulance services, hospitals, nursing homes, home care agencies, social service agencies, public health departments . . . all of them have seen what aggressive behavior can do to the healthcare professional, and, sadly, some episodes have had catastrophic outcomes.

Dealing with an issue as sensitive as aggression management can be difficult, and many questions are presented when this topic is explored. What rights does the provider have in protecting him- or herself? To what extent can a provider defend him- or herself? Is it ethical for a healthcare provider to take aggressive actions to avoid becoming a victim? There are no easy answers to these questions. Each provider must look inside him- or herself for answers. Legal counsel may provide safe information to prevent criminal prosecution or to fend off civil litigation, but the provider must still be comfortable with his or her choice.

The causes of aggressive behavior are numerous. Often aggressive behavior is secondary to some form of drug or alcohol abuse. Although we may frequently encounter this type of aggression, we cannot forget that there are many causes, including mental health diseases, metabolic disorders, head injuries, chemical exposure, and a host of others. For the purposes of this text, the cause is not critical. Regardless of the reason behind the violence, the provider still has to be able to protect him- or herself, not only for personal safety and survival, but also to continue to provide quality care.

In this text, the terms *prehospital provider, healthcare provider,* and *caregiver* are frequently used. It is important to understand the difference in terminology, so proper association may be made with the content. Prehospital providers are those professionals who provide emergency medical treatment prior to a patient's arrival to a hospital. Commonly, these are EMTs and paramedics. Healthcare providers are those professionals who provide healthcare services in a more structured setting, such as hospitals, nursing homes, and clinics. Caregiver refers to any provider, regardless of where the care is given or in what manner it is provided. This would include prehospital providers, healthcare providers, and others involved in the delivery of health services, such as midwives, home care providers, aides, and technicians.

This text is intended to help prepare the healthcare professional to deal with aggressive behavior. It is not about "fighting." It is about *surviving.* We have spent most of our adult lives as healthcare professionals dealing with virtually every form of aggression and violence. Our backgrounds are unique, complement each other, and encompass all aspects of health care including prehospital care, acute care, psychiatric care, home care, and long-term care. The methods of dealing with aggressive behavior that are presented in this text are not based on idealistic suppositions. Instead, they are based on experience, research, and practice. Every method introduced has been tried with success. It is not our intention that you read this book and consider yourself well versed in aggression management; we encourage you to treat it like every other clinical skill you've learned. Successful de-escalation of aggressive behavior is an art that requires practice, rehearsal, and evaluation.

Steve Wilder and Chris Sorensen

About the Authors

Steve Wilder, CHSP, EMT-P

Steve Wilder has spent the past 17 years practicing healthcare risk management in acute care hospitals, outpatient surgery centers, small rural hospitals, and long-term care facilities. Mr. Wilder has developed management programs in the Safety, Life Safety, Hazardous Materials, Security, and Emergency Preparedness sections of the Joint Commission on the Accreditation of Healthcare Organizations (JCAHO) Environment of Care. Originally the founder of S. Wilder and Associates, Inc., he has been a consultant for hospitals and nursing homes in the areas of safety, security, and risk management program administration since 1990.

An experienced trial expert, Mr. Wilder has consulted for several law firms and insurance companies on issues of healthcare safety and risk management. He also has written numerous articles for magazines and trade journals.

In addition to his career in healthcare risk management, Mr. Wilder has also spent the past 23 years in the fire service, currently holding the rank of deputy chief. He is an Illinois-licensed paramedic, a certified fire science instructor, and on the teaching staff for the University of Illinois Fire Service Institute and at Southern Illinois University. He has written one book on fire service risk management and has been involved in the production of over twenty videos on healthcare safety, security, and risk management.

Mr. Wilder earned his bachelor's degree in business administration from Governor's State University in University Park, Illinois. He also holds teaching certificates in numerous areas of public safety administration. In addition, he has attained the master level as a Certified Healthcare Safety Professional.

Chris Sorensen, CHPA

Chris Sorensen has spent 20 years in healthcare safety and security management at some of the largest, most prestigious healthcare organizations in the country. Mr. Sorensen has served as the Chief Safety Officer with responsibility for all seven areas of the JCAHO Environment of Care, developing management programs in the Safety, Life Safety, Hazardous Materials, Security, Medical Equipment, Utilities, and Emergency Preparedness sections of the Environment of Care. After joining S. Wilder & Associates, Inc., in 1992 as a consultant, Mr. Sorensen became a partner with the firm in 1996, when the name was changed to Sorensen, Wilder and Associates (SWA). Through SWA, he has consulted for hospitals, nursing homes, government agencies, retailing, and industry in areas of safety and security management.

A recognized expert in the field of hospital security, Mr. Sorensen has been actively involved in numerous professional organizations impacting healthcare safety and security services, including:

- International Association of Healthcare Security & Safety (IAHSS), serving as chairman for the Chicago Chapter of IAHSS
- American Society of Industrial Security (ASIS)
- Illinois Security Chiefs Association (ISCA)
- Police Self Defense Instructors International, serving as Illinois State Director and Midwest Regional Director

Mr. Sorensen achieved IAHSS's highest recognition in 1994, Certified Healthcare Protection Administrator (CHPA). He is also a martial artist and has trained thousands of police officers, security officers, physicians, nurses, paramedics, and EMTs across the nation in self-defense and defensive tactics. He has written and directed over thirty videos on health-care safety and security management.

Mr. Sorensen is published in a variety of books, training films, and newsletters on topics related to public safety.

Foreword

Violence in America has spilled over into the workplace, putting at risk the personal safety, productivity, and mental and physical health of American workers. According to data provided by the U.S. Department of Justice and the Bureau of Justice Statistics, violence in the workplace is now at epidemic levels. The U.S. Department of Justice[1] reports that incidents of workplace violence now exceed one million a year, with the most common type being simple assault. Healthcare workers continue to be some of the leading victims of violent acts against workers.

There are many causes of workplace violence—economic, societal, psychological, and organizational. The 1990s were filled with economic compressions, overstressed populations, downsizing and rightsizing of organizations, massive layoffs, growth and technology changes, recessions, and mergers and acquisitions. When these are added to societal concerns such as increased accessibility of handguns and the portrayal of violence as an acceptable means of dealing with life stresses in movies, television shows, and music, one begins to see the mosaic of external forces that could have a role in episodes of workplace violence.

While one would think that acts of workplace violence are unpredictable and nonpreventable, the security industry reports that violence in the workplace is, in fact, both predictable and preventable. The key to predicting and preventing workplace violence is to prepare for it, recognize it, and intervene appropriately. The content of this book will provide you with the necessary tools to do so.

The primary mission of this book is to provide an operational resource for healthcare professionals who find themselves concerned about workplace violence and want to better manage such situations. The content is based on practical applications, as opposed to theoretical concepts, which goes to the very heart of the importance of this book. In the complexity and variety of workplace violence situations for which this book prepares individuals; one must not forget to evaluate every incident independently. In that vein, this book is not intended to be the total, final, or best answer to all incidents that arise. Rather, it presents possible solutions and multiple approaches to situations, as well as information of which individuals in the healthcare environment should be aware, keeping in mind that incidents must be considered on a case-by-case basis.

Clearly, there are no easy or simple answers in dealing with workplace violence situations, but this book gives you the closest thing possible to such answers. How to begin and then continue to be educated and prepared for workplace violence is found in the pages of this book. Although having to deal with a workplace violence situation in health care may be an event that people believe will never happen to them, the reality is that healthcare workers have a high exposure rate. Preparedness as we begin the new millennium includes recognizing and responding to this threat.

Monica C. Berry, RN, JD, FASHRM
Chicago, Illinois

---

[1]www.svn.net/mikekell/v6.html

Acknowledgments

We would like to thank the following people for their contributions to the success of this project:

Dr. John Moran
Communicorp Inc.
Lombard, Illinois

Ryland Gagnon
Precision Video and Photography
Bradley, Illinois

Chris "Bubba" Capuzzi
Obsession Tattoos
Bradley, Illinois

Jeff Brosseau, EMT-P
Linda Bruno, RN
Provena St. Mary's Trauma Center
Kankakee, Illinois

Chief Leon Fritz
Capt. Greg Glidewell
Bradley, Illinois Fire Department

Essentials of Aggression Management in Health Care

The Impact of Violence on Prehospital Providers

The Jeff Cook Story

February 13, 1998, was much the same as any other day for Lt. Jeff Cook of the Toledo, Ohio, Fire Department. Assigned to Engine 18, normally averaging nine runs per shift, Lt. Cook had responded to four calls for assistance that day. None of them were out of the ordinary. The drill for the day was a confined space rescue. Soon, what started as just another "call for service" would change Lt. Cook's life forever.

At 1555 hours, Toledo dispatch assigned Engine 18 to 1358 Brookpark to help the Lifesquad on a call for multiple stabbing victims. Upon arrival, Lt. Cook assumed command and began directing operations. Police were on the scene, and management of the incident was as "routine" as one would expect a multiple trauma run to be. Dr. Ed San Miguel responded from St. Vincent Hospital, which is the response protocol for the Toledo Fire Department on all multiple casualty incidents. Dr. San Miguel assumed management of the patients. At the scene, a 27-year-old female was in traumatic arrest due to multiple stab wounds from an unknown perpetrator. The perpetrator also stabbed her 10-year-old son in the stomach and slashed her 12-year-old daughter several times on various parts of her body. In addition, the family's pets, two cats and a dog, were unmercifully stabbed to death.

To allow paramedics to treat the traumatic arrest patient, Lt. Cook drove the Lifesquad to the Toledo hospital. Another Lifesquad, also operating at the scene, had already departed for the hospital, with Lt. Cook and his crew leaving shortly afterward. For safety, Lt. Cook stayed several car lengths behind the first Lifesquad, which allowed him to see the traffic patterns of other vehicles and pedestrians. While traveling south on Jackman Road, Lt. Cook saw a male standing in the road, holding what appeared to be a stick. He then observed the subject raise the "stick" he now recognized as a shotgun, firing a shot directly at the Lifesquad ahead of him. Realizing what was happening, Lt. Cook accelerated his ambulance, with the intent of running down the armed offender, who by now had fired two shots into the lead Lifesquad. Before Lt. Cook could get to him, the offender jumped into a van and drove off, cutting through a service station lot to escape.

After radioing for help and observing the offender drive off, Lt. Cook pulled up beside the disabled Lifesquad unit. Lt. Cook exited his vehicle and ran to the aid of his comrade. He opened the driver's door and found him lying on the floor, between the seats. His foot was still pressed against the brake pedal. Placing the Lifesquad in park, Lt. Cook assessed the driver, who had sustained facial lacerations caused by the shattering glass. Walking around to the other side of the Lifesquad, Lt. Cook unexpectedly found himself confronted by the perpetrator. Now, with only 14 feet separating the two of them, Lt. Cook stood face-to-face with the individual who had just fired upon his partners in an attempt to end their lives, and who was about to attempt to take his. Lt. Cook would later learn that this was the same individual who stabbed the victims he and his crews were treating. Looking at the attacker, Lt. Cook saw a smile spread across his face, a smirk he will remember and visualize for the rest of his life. Lt. Cook then saw the barrel of a shotgun pointing directly at him. Realizing that he had nowhere to run, Lt. Cook saw his life pass before him. In a split second, the world and the career that Lt. Jeff Cook knew and loved were senselessly snatched away from him, perhaps forever.

It played out like a slow-motion nightmare. The blast from the 12-gauge shotgun, the discharge of the pellets, increasingly painful upon impact, tearing into his left arm, effortlessly ripped the flesh from his bones. Finding himself on the ground, still stunned from the events and the traumatic injuries, Lt. Cook managed to find his portable radio. He contacted his dispatcher and gave a description of the fleeing van and the license plate number. Only then did he remember to tell them he was shot and needed assistance.

At the time, even Lt. Cook did not realize how serious his injuries were. Thirty-one pellets from the blast entered his body. Besides the twenty-four that caused his arm injuries, which included a crushed humerus, radius, and ulna, one pellet entered his chest cavity, penetrating his lung. Another one entered his stomach, and five more grazed his back. As his own crew placed him in the ambulance, Lt. Cook lost consciousness and would remain comatose for the next two days. Later, he discovered that the perpetrator who shot him at point-blank range fled the scene, abandoned his van, and attempted to hijack a truck from a 21-year-old pregnant female. When she refused to surrender her truck, he shot her in the back, killing her and her unborn child. With police pursuing, the individual fled in a stolen van, firing shots into the pursuing squad car. Police finally forced him into a spin and were able to stop him in a grocery store parking lot. Exiting the stolen van, the offender was shot and killed by police. Miraculously, no bystanders were injured at the scene, although seven cars were hit by gunfire.

In the emergency department, the physicians diagnosed Lt. Cook with multiple traumatic injuries that resulted in two open sucking chest wounds, a tension pneumothorax, and a hemothorax. After two days in a comatose state, Lt. Cook slowly began to regain consciousness. As he awakened, his first memory was seeing his daughter, Ashley, who had turned eight years old the day after the shooting. Holding onto his finger, she simply said, "Papa, I love you" when she saw his eyes open. Lt. Jeff Cook then realized that he was alive and that he had a very good reason for battling his way back to good health. Still, he knew the road to recovery was not going to be an easy one to travel.

Lt. Cook spent seven more days in the intensive care unit before being discharged to his parents' care. There he spent the next four months, receiving physical therapy treatments daily. He has undergone four surgeries so far to repair his physical injuries. But despite his physical progression, no physician has been able to surgically remove the emotional scars that continue to be a part of his life.

On November 15, 1998, Lt. Jeff Cook returned to work in a modified duty capacity. Unable to fight fires, he was assigned to a supervisory position in the

Toledo Fire Alarm office. While he is happy to be working, he is not satisfied with his current position. "I'm a firefighter," Jeff says. "It's who I am. It's the job I love, the greatest job in the world. Now, I have to sit in the office and send firefighters and prehospital personnel on runs . . . I miss it." His words fade off into a silent ending. His feelings are sincere. His pain runs deeper than we can imagine.

A year later, many physical injuries have healed. However, the emotional scars remain open and deep. "I am sick of being sick," he says. A left-hander, Lt. Cook has very limited mobility and use of his left wrist. Although he cannot explain why, he now dislikes being in crowds and goes to great lengths to avoid people he doesn't know. Furthermore, he worries about how this will affect his health later in life. "At 44 years old, I am forced to start my life over." While he says he has grown closer to friends and family as a result of the tragedy, he still has trouble being alone. He also admits to having to medicate himself both to get to sleep and to avoid the horrible nightmares.

He also asks "Why?"—a question he knows will never be answered. When the police killed the gunman, they forever sealed all answers in a vault of speculation. "I wish I knew why he did this, why he turned on the rescue workers, and why he came back for us. We will never know. We never expected this to happen to us. We are all used to people appreciating us and the help we give. It's always the police involved in shootings. The fire department is not prepared for gunfights."

• • • • • • • • • •

Could anything have been done to prevent this catastrophe from occurring? Probably not. Lt. Jeff Cook and his crew were in the wrong place at the wrong time, and he is paying the price.

Because of this incident, the Toledo Fire Department now stages all equipment and manpower so that police are on the scene first to determine whether the environment is safe and secure.

We wish Lt. Jeff Cook and all of his brothers with the Toledo Fire Department nothing but the best as they continue to recover from this nightmare. We hope none of us ever again go through what these individuals have endured.

Stay safe, and Godspeed.

Introduction

Ask any long-term emergency medical care provider about the changes in society during their years of service. Most will tell you there has been an increase in violent behavior in society over the past two or three decades. In the 1970s, violence against prehospital providers was rare or unreported. People in need of emergency medical care appreciated the presence of prehospital providers and saw it as a sign of professional help and hope for a positive outcome. When prehospital providers arrived on the scene, others at the scene would normally clear a path to allow the providers access and room to treat the patient. At that time, prehospital providers were truly considered "the good guys in the white hats."

The mid and late 1980s saw a transition begin to take place. Violence became more prevalent in our society. During this time we began to see an

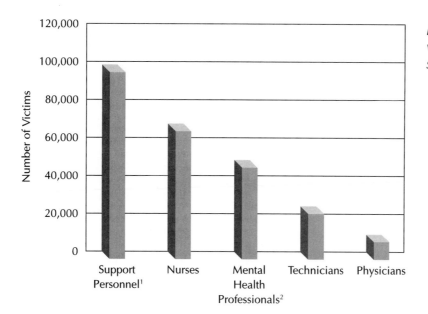

Figure 1-1 *Victims of nonfatal workplace violence in health care.*

Source: U.S. Bureau of Labor Statistics, 1996

[1]Support Personnel includes security officers, nurse's aides, transporters, etc.
[2]Mental Health Professionals include physicians, nurses, and technicians
  that work in mental health institutions.

increase in the number of violent incidents to which prehospital providers were responding. Forms of violence previously unheard of or seldom discussed were suddenly becoming commonplace in American society.

The 1990s seemed to become the decade for violent behavior. Sadly, violence in our society is now a common event. The news media brings to our attention new incidents of violence that once shocked and appalled us but now leave us often without emotion or empathy.

It is a sad state to be living in a society in which violence is so commonplace and accepted. Even sadder is that this violence often affects those who are called upon to help the victims. Most prehospital providers with any degree of longevity can identify or recall at least one incident in which they were the victim of violent or aggressive behavior at the hands of a patient. When called upon to provide emergency medical care for the victim of a violent crime, prehospital providers potentially find themselves in the middle of violent behavior. Prehospital providers should never forget: *When you are called into a situation where violence has occurred, there is an increased potential for more violence to occur, with you as the victim.*

Unfortunately, this also holds true for hospital emergency departments, mental health departments, and other hospital units. Regardless of socioeconomic class, type of patient, scenario, time of day, or other factors, the potential for violence extends into the hospital. Much like prehospital providers, hospital providers must recognize the risk and be prepared in advance to deal with it.

The Prehospital Provider and Domestic Violence

How severe is the problem of violence in our communities today? Violence in the workplace is a direct manifestation of increasing violence in our society. Few people realize that violence in the workplace is the leading cause of fatal occupational injuries among women (OSHA, 1996).

According to the Occupational Safety and Health Administration (OSHA, 1996), incidents of violence resulting in the death and injury of healthcare and community workers have occurred in emergency departments, psychiatric units, mental health clinics, social service agencies, and home healthcare services at an alarming rate over the past few years. These settings saw an increase in assaults, hostage taking, sexual assaults, robbery, and other violent actions. Why are these statistics and facts of concern to prehospital providers? Think about any random act of violence occurring in your community. Regardless of the type of injury, mechanism of injury, or scenario, prehospital providers will be called to respond. In responding, prehospital providers may find themselves in the middle of potentially aggressive behavior. Suddenly the rescuer becomes the victim.

Why is it that in the past two decades we have seen an increase in violence in our society? Certainly the increase in domestic violence across the nation plays a leading role. Domestic violence crosses ethnic, racial, age, national origin, sexual orientation, religious, social, and economic lines. In a 1995 report, the U.S. Bureau of Justice Statistics estimated that every year more than one million women are victims of nonfatal violence at the hands of an acquaintance. In a similar report, the American Psychological Association (1996) found that nearly one in three adult women will experience at least one physical assault at the hands of an adult partner at some point in her life.

Who are the victims of domestic violence? According to the U.S. Bureau of Justice Statistics (1995), 90% to 95% of all acts of domestic violence are against women, with the majority of victims between the ages of 19 and 29. Not surprisingly, as many as 95% of domestic violence perpetrators are male. In addition, male perpetrators are four times more likely to use lethal violence than are their female counterparts. Prehospital providers must realize they are responsible for recognizing early warnings of domestic violence and for reporting these situations to the proper authorities in the emergency department.

The rate of domestic violence detection by emergency department providers is low. One article in the *Journal of the American Medical Association* suggests battered women may comprise 20% to 30% of ambulatory care patients seen in emergency departments (Hyman et al., 1995). However, medical practitioners only identify one in twenty as being a victim of domestic violence. Sadly, the same study found that less than 3% of women visiting the emergency department disclose that they are victims of domestic violence. Additionally, nurses and physicians rarely ask about domestic violence. Finally, the same study found that "acute domestic violence" was the reason for one of nine emergency department visits among women with a current partner.

Prehospital providers may be recognized as a mechanism for detecting domestic and other forms of violence. Still, one question must be answered first. Should we place prehospital providers in the role of "policing" for violence? Obviously, providing quality medical care to the patient should remain their first concern. When faced with a domestic violence situation, a prehospital provider must consider removing the patient from the environment in which the violence may have taken place. Often, the patient who is the victim of aggression may not feel comfortable talking about it while in the same room, or building, where it took place. Once moved to a safer environment, the patient may willingly provide more specific information.

When faced with such a situation, prehospital providers have several choices available to them. The first (and least preferred) action the prehospital provider may take is to confront and question the person alleged to have committed the violence. Except in communities where police officers also provide prehospital services, this option is not considered viable. The prehospital provider could conceivably compromise his or her own personal safety or take action that could later compromise criminal prosecution. Another option is to report the incident to local law enforcement. Although a safer alternative for the prehospital provider, this option is not free from risk. Police officers are trained in law enforcement. Their intentions may be noble, but unless they receive special training to deal with victims of violent crime, they may not be as effective as one would hope. Additionally, because of the authority they represent and their power to incarcerate or detain offenders, police officers may intimidate the victim. For a variety of reasons, the victim may fear seeing the offender incarcerated. As a result, the victim may not provide the police officer with a factual representation of how the incident occurred.

Dr. Joseph R. Danna is project medical director for the EMS system at Provena St. Mary's Hospital in Kankakee, Illinois. Over the past few years, Dr. Danna has become a leader in Illinois for his ongoing effort to train and prepare emergency service workers in recognizing and dealing with the increased domestic violence in our society. As project medical director, Dr. Danna prefers that prehospital providers in his system observe conditions at the scene and communicate them to the medical staff in the emergency department. For prehospital providers, incidents of domestic violence in the field are to be dealt with like any other form of needed emergency medical care. They are the eyes and ears for the emergency department physician. They should make an assessment of this situation as they would in any other and report their observations to the physician in the emergency department. Special training provided for nurses and physicians in the emergency department allows them to deal with the victim in nonintimidating, nonthreatening ways. They are also able to make a better determination of the circumstances and surroundings in which the victim lives. Additionally, while providing nonthreatening intervention, physicians and nurses are often able to help victims of domestic violence escape their fear-filled environment.

The OSHA Workplace Violence Standard

The increase in violence in our society is indisputable. Healthcare professionals drawn into the middle of this violence must receive special training just as they do for any other hazardous environment. The U.S. Department of Labor, through the Occupational Safety and Health Administration, recently introduced OSHA 3148, "Guidelines for Preventing Workplace Violence for Healthcare and Social Service Workers." This standard, designed to help healthcare organizations prepare for increased exposure to workplace violence, is clearly written to include prehospital providers.

Commonly referred to as the OSHA Workplace Violence Standard, the act is still in draft form, not yet signed into law. Still, OSHA uses the basic content of this act as a tool of enforcement under its General Duty Clause. Under the General Duty Clause, when an unsafe act or condition exists that the employer knew about or should have known about, OSHA may enforce monetary penalties, regardless of the absence of a specific standard.

As written, the OSHA Workplace Violence Standard is divided into five parts:

1. Management Commitment and Employee Involvement
2. A Worksite Analysis/Risk Assessment
3. Development of Hazard Prevention and Controls
4. Training
5. Recordkeeping

Each of these areas contains specific criteria that OSHA requires the employer (and employee) to meet to be considered compliant.

Management Commitment and Employee Involvement

Management commitment is an often misunderstood and misperceived component of the program. Commitment and involvement by all levels of management are critical to the success of the program. However, commitment means more than generating memorandums and making statements in newsletters. Management commitment includes providing the organization with the resources necessary to perform a qualified risk assessment. Additionally, employers must provide staff with the proper tools and the time and resources to obtain training by competent and qualified instructors.

Management also shows its concern for the employees' health and safety by placing a high priority on programs and processes designed to lessen the risk of injury in the workplace. Considering the extreme risk prehospital providers are placed at when performing their duties, management commitment to a workplace violence prevention program is essential.

Top management must develop a written plan for recognizing the risk of violence against prehospital providers as an occupational hazard. They must also place the employees' health and safety on the same level of importance as patients'. The implementation of the policy requires management to integrate all issues and aspects of employee health and safety concerns into daily operating procedures, thereby lessening the risk of injury. (See sample written plan at the end of this chapter.)

In the written plan, the organization should also commit to providing a violence-free environment for all employees. There is a difference between "committing" to providing an environment free from the risk of violence and "striving" to provide an environment that is free from violence. An organization that "commits" to providing an environment free of the risk of violence falls short of their commitment and goal every time a violent incident occurs. An organization that "strives" to provide an environment that is free from risk of violence succeeds with every shift change without an incident of violence. From a risk management and loss exposure perspective, the organization must exercise due regard for the terminology used in the development of its workplace violence prevention policy.

In addition to the commitments and obligations of management, employees owe themselves something. For a violence prevention program to be successful, employee involvement is critical. Areas of employee involvement may include the following:

- Understanding and complying with the department or agency's workplace violence prevention program (as well as all other safety policies).
- An employee suggestion or complaint process allowing employees to communicate concerns to management and to receive feedback without fear of reprisal or consequence.

- A system designed and implemented to ensure reporting of incidents that place the employee at risk of violent behavior. Such a system must include appropriate incident report forms, reporting mechanisms, investigative processes, and appropriate follow-up to be successful.
- A functional safety committee should exist in the organization that regularly addresses the topic of workplace violence against the prehospital provider. Organization employees should have access to the safety committee. They should also be able to provide feedback and information, allowing the safety committee to perform its duties more effectively. The safety committee must share actions and information with the employees regularly.

When incidents of violence against prehospital providers occur, staff must complete appropriate documentation and provide essential follow-up. Employees should participate in some type of case conference or other periodic reviews to identify contributing and precipitating events that led to the violent behavior. This information, used effectively, provides resources for future training materials. Employees must participate in training programs designed to help them prepare for potential aggressive behavior.

Finally, the organization must have a written program that includes the elements identified previously and any other elements determined essential by the organization. Management must provide the written program to all organizational employees. Additionally, management needs to review the program with staff and offer them the opportunity to question and clarify key points of the program.

The written program should include the following, at minimum:

- A zero tolerance policy created by and disseminated throughout the organization. This policy should include physical violence, verbal abuse, nonverbal abuse, and other similar actions. (See sample zero tolerance policy at the end of this chapter.)
- Assurance that no reprisals will be taken against any employee who reports experiencing or witnessing incidents of workplace violence.
- Encouragement for employees to report any form of workplace violence as soon as it happens.
- A comprehensive plan for dealing with known conditions that have a greater risk of violence than other scenarios commonly encountered.
- Assigned responsibility and authority to individuals or teams.

A Worksite Analysis/Risk Assessment

A complete worksite analysis is the first step in conducting a risk assessment. The worksite analysis identifies unsafe conditions that may increase the likelihood of or contribute to the risk of violent or aggressive behavior against the prehospital provider. Unlike a worksite analysis performed at a fixed location, such as in a hospital emergency department, the worksite analysis for prehospital care must include many different scenarios and possibilities. The prehospital worksite analysis may include the following:

- A complete review of emergency "run sheets" to identify patients who have demonstrated patterns of aggressive behavior against police officers, prehospital providers, firefighters, or other emergency service personnel. Used productively, this information may assist in preventing future recurrence of aggressive acts against prehospital providers. Still, the prehospital provider should never compromise a patient's right to medical confidentiality.

- Identification and analysis of any apparent trends in aggressive actions against prehospital providers. Factors may include day of the week, time of day, specific environments, specific locations, etc. Documentation may also include underlying information such as threats to prehospital providers prior to the aggressive acts or the identification or classification of patients likely to be aggressive.
- Identification of scenarios in which staff is at an increased risk of violence.
- A checklist for use by emergency dispatchers in preassessing the risk of violence. The dispatcher communicates the findings to prehospital providers en route to a call. This information allows the prehospital providers to prepare for potentially aggressive behavior prior to arrival.
- Use of restricted duty positions to keep injured prehospital providers in the workplace and return them to regular, productive, full-time status as quickly and safely as possible.
- Analysis of equipment carried by prehospital providers used to restrain or control aggressive patients in an emergency situation.
- Assessment of new vehicles and apparatus used to provide care and treatment to patients, including those who may be potentially violent. Management should design apparatus to simplify gaining physical control of the patient. For example, prehospital providers should be able to control the patient's behavior without physically placing themselves over the patient and in harm's way due to cramped or restricted positioning.

Development of Hazard Prevention and Controls

Unlike emergency departments, psychiatric units, and outpatient clinics, where doctors and nurses provide care to patients in a controlled setting, the prehospital provider provides emergency medical care in a variety of settings that are often much less controlled. These may include medical facilities, industrial settings, residential settings, office environments, city streets and sidewalks, or rural areas remote from other people or amenities. Emergency medical care may be provided in a fixed setting or in the back of a moving ambulance. Implementing engineering controls designed to prevent violence or lessen the impact of violence in fixed settings such as emergency departments is much less challenging than implementing those intended for use in the prehospital setting.

Engineering Controls for Prehospital Care

Engineering controls refers to the physical environment in which an individual performs his or her duties or functions. Addressing engineering controls for prehospital providers is difficult. Despite this challenge, there are certain engineering controls that can be evaluated and acted upon to increase the safety of prehospital providers treating an aggressive patient. These may include the following items.

Ambulance Design
Any prehospital provider who has ever attempted to perform techniques of physical aggression control or patient restraint in the back of an ambulance will tell you that the patient often has the distinct advantage. In many

ambulances, design specifications are such that the patient cot sits flush against a side wall. As a result, the prehospital provider who is attempting to control the aggressive patient is only able to approach the patient from one side. This is one argument in favor of designing ambulances so the stretcher locks in place in the center of the floor, allowing the prehospital provider access to the patient from both sides of the patient. Hence, a prehospital provider is able to provide clinical care while safely restraining and controlling a patient's behavior during periods of aggression.

Cabinet or compartment layout is also a concern when designing ambulances. Cabinets are often out of the way. A prehospital provider must often stand and find equipment in overhead compartments or, worse, reach across a patient. Compartments need to be located where they provide quick, unobstructed access, maximizing safety for the patient and the provider.

Prehospital providers must also consider accessibility to the patient compartment of the ambulance by family members or friends a potential risk. In violent or potentially violent environments, the prehospital provider must be able to secure and protect himself and his patient quickly, including preventing access by unauthorized outsiders.

Safety Equipment

Prehospital providers may also use equipment designed for patient safety to protect themselves. Almost every patient cot has some form of safety restraint device for the patient. In many cases, patient cots are equipped with either two or three safety belts, and in some cases, a shoulder harness belt system is provided as well. These systems designed for patient safety during transportation, when properly applied, also offer a limited degree of safety to the prehospital provider. In cases in which the patient shows signs of aggressive behavior toward the prehospital provider, the presence of safety belts may allow the prehospital provider a quick source for restraining a patient. Additionally, it may allow the prehospital provider a few extra moments to defend against an attack.

Patient Restraint Devices

In Chapter 9, we will look at various types of restraint devices common to prehospital emergency medical care and their intended use. In addition, we will discuss the legal considerations of restraining a patient. Used appropriately, patient restraint devices become an engineering tool. Fortunately for prehospital providers, patient restraint devices are seldom needed. Therefore, it is imperative for prehospital providers to regularly check patient restraint devices to ensure proper working condition and readiness.

Soft Body Armor (Bulletproof Vests)

In high risk/high crime areas, the use of bulletproof vests by prehospital providers is not uncommon. Unfortunately, such an investment is often seen as impractical until after an incident occurs. Then, in a truly reactive mode, the department finds itself scurrying to take steps to make certain that repeat incidents do not take place.

Based on a comprehensive risk assessment, bulletproof vests and other such "uncommon" protective devices should be considered and provided as necessary.

Portable Radios

Critical to safety is the ability to assess a situation, perform a quick risk assessment (sizeup), and be able to notify a dispatch center when help is needed. Sitting in the cab of an ambulance with an installed radio system readily available makes this much easier to accomplish. Working in an area remote from the ambulance is another story.

Every prehospital provider working in the field needs to have some form of communication available in the event urgent help is needed. In many agencies, portable radios (walkie-talkies) are supplied for the prehospital provider. While the availability of the portable radio is essential, other elements must also be considered:

- Does the portable radio have sufficient power to transmit a signal from anywhere the prehospital provider may be providing service?
- Is the base station staffed and monitored around the clock, assuring that someone will always answer the call for help?
- Does the prehospital provider have channel priority, or is the channel shared with other police, fire, or business users?
- Is there a procedure in place to ensure that the battery in the radio is fully charged and functional at the start of and throughout each shift?
- Is there a well-documented and rehearsed coded message system in place that the prehospital provider can use when he or she cannot easily or safely discuss the entire situation over the radio?

Work Practice Controls for Prehospital Care

When addressing the environment that prehospital providers work in, we address engineering controls. When we address work practice controls, we are addressing *how* people do their jobs. Engineering controls alone offer limited effectiveness. Work practice controls must be included for any program to be effective in maximizing safety to the prehospital provider.

Following are some of the work practice controls that should be given consideration.

Uniforms

Uniforms should be designed in such a way that they allow the prehospital provider freedom of movement and freedom from risk of injury. While many departments prefer badges, name tags, and collar insignias to be affixed to the uniform, these articles are often secured with a pin. Combative patients can easily use these pins as sharp weapons against the prehospital provider.

For a variety of reasons many organizations and systems require the prehospital provider to carry a backup set of keys to the ambulance. While this is practical, the prehospital provider must consider that keys make an excellent weapon when they fall into the wrong hands. Uniforms, including carried articles, should be designed in such a way that required tools and equipment are not openly visible to the aggressive patient.

Instrument pouches are another serious concern when addressing prehospital provider safety. Many prehospital providers carry a variety of scissors, forceps, hemostats, etc., on their belt or in their pouch. While preparedness is essential in managing the emergency needs of the patient, many of these same articles make excellent weapons when they fall into the hands of an aggressive patient. If prehospital providers are going to carry tool pouches, the pouch should be designed with a protective cover to prevent accidental dropping or unintentional removal of the pouch contents.

Teamwork

Dealing with an aggressive patient presents unique risks to the prehospital provider. This risk is greatly intensified when prehospital providers find themselves alone with an aggressive patient. If it is true that there is safety in numbers, then certainly the odds of being injured at the hands of an aggressive patient are much less when working in teams. If your patient shows signs of aggressive behavior (Chapter 4 will address an aggression continuum), it is critical for your safety and well-being that you always stay with a partner. If additional help is necessary, one of the prehospital providers should use the portable radio rather than leave the room or the building to make the call. If it is necessary for one prehospital provider to leave the room or building, both prehospital providers should leave.

Police Department Liaison

Usually, police officers or other law enforcement agencies can quickly and easily identify high-risk areas. Dispatchers frequently send officers to these locations for a variety of reasons. The use of a liaison between the prehospital agency and the local police department is an effective tool in helping prehospital providers identify high-risk areas or addresses. Additionally, this becomes an excellent opportunity to utilize dual dispatches, so that both police and emergency medical services are mobilized at the same time and hopefully arrive at the scene within moments of each other.

Training

Training and education are key components in ensuring that all staff is aware of potential risks before finding themselves in potentially violent situations. Every prehospital provider receives training in protection from exposure to blood and body fluids and the use of universal precautions in preventing exposures. This concept of universal precautions can be used in preventing exposure to violence as well. Training programs are designed to enable the prehospital provider to recognize potentially violent situations before they develop and to prepare to deal with them in a proactive manner as opposed to reactive.

Annual training should be provided to all employees who may find themselves at risk of exposure to violent situations as a result of their employment. At minimum, these training programs should include:

- Review of the agency's workplace violence prevention policy
- Risk factors that cause or contribute to violent episodes
- Early recognition of progressive aggressive behavior
- The stages of aggression
- Aggression/de-escalation techniques
- Cultural diversity awareness
- Dealing with hostile bystanders
- Behavior control methods
- Safe application of restraint devices
- Use of the buddy system for personal protection
- Escapes from grabs and holds*
- Blocking techniques*
- Basic takedown techniques*
- Basic holds*
- Reporting requirements
- Procedures for obtaining medical (physical and/or emotional) assistance after an incident

(*Note:* Those marked with an asterisk (*) should only be learned from a qualified self-defense instructor and are only to be used in cases in which the use of force can be justified to protect oneself from injury or death. Prehospital providers must be aware of the laws on the use of force in their respective jurisdictions.)

Recordkeeping

Recordkeeping is an essential part of the success of any program. In addition to meeting recordkeeping requirements that may be mandated by federal or state agencies, the department will quickly learn that good recordkeeping is the basis for identifying opportunities for improvement in their program.

The following records are among those to be considered important.

OSHA Log of Injury or Illness (OSHA 200 Log)

OSHA requires an entry on the OSHA 200 log whenever an occupational injury occurs and meets any of the following conditions:

- Requires treatment that is "greater than first aid"
- Results in lost time
- Results in restricted or modified "light duty"
- Results in loss of consciousness
- Causes death

In addition, if the injury results in a fatality or in the hospitalization of three or more employees (including emergency room treatment), *then the regional OSHA office must be notified within eight hours of the incident.* (*Note:* In some states OSHA laws do not apply to governmental agencies, therefore, prehospital providers in governmental agencies such as fire departments may not be bound by these reporting requirements. Verification should be made with the regional OSHA office or the labor department in the state that has jurisdiction.)

Medical Reports

Any time an employee is assaulted, the incident should be investigated and a file established. Medical records of work injuries should be included in the documentation, but in such a way that the employee's right to medical confidentiality is not compromised. Many agencies maintain an employee health file for all employee health records, including those related to injuries sustained on the job. In this practice, the records are separate from other employee files and allow a greater degree of confidentiality and protection. Access to these records should be controlled and restricted to the organization's risk manager, human resource manager, or other designated representative.

Medical reports related to workplace violence should include at minimum the circumstances leading up to the incident, the injuries sustained, the action taken, and any other circumstances related to the incident.

Incident Reports

The agency needs some type of incident report that can be used to document any situation, event, or circumstance that is out of the ordinary for that agency. This incident report becomes an administrative tool that can be used to help identify unplanned or unexpected events that occur and to analyze any trend these events may represent to better prepare for future recurrences. The department or agency's safety committee or similar team should review incident reports that relate to violent incidents involving prehospital providers. As these reports are reviewed, the department's violence prevention program can be updated as necessary for maximum efficacy.

Summary

We live in a society that seems to turn to violence to solve problems. As long as man's inhumanity to others continues to play out in our homes and businesses and on our streets, prehospital providers will continue to be called into action. In every case, the prehospital provider potentially becomes the victim of the next aggressive act.

Prehospital agencies can take steps to protect their employees by being proactive in the following ways:

1. Committing to providing an environment that is as free from risk of violence as is possible
2. Conducting qualified worksite analysis and risk assessments to determine where prehospital providers are at greatest risk of violence
3. Developing engineering controls and work practice controls to maximize safety for the prehospital provider in the field
4. Providing ongoing training to prehospital providers in all areas of aggression management and behavior control techniques
5. Documenting all incidents of violent behavior and using documentation records to develop new preventive programs and to improve existing programs.

References

American Psychological Association. (1996). Violence in the Family: Report of the American Psychological Association Presidential Task Force on Violence and the Family. Washington, DC: Government Printing Office.

Hyman et al. (June 1995). "Laws Mandating Reporting of Domestic Violence: Do They Promote Patient Well-Being?" *Journal of the American Medical Association.* Vol. 273, No. 22, 1781.

Occupational Safety and Health Administration (OSHA). (1996). OSHA Workplace Violence Awareness and Prevention Facts and Information. Fact Sheet No. OSHA 96-53. www.osha.gov.

U.S. Department of Justice, Bureau of Justice Statistics. (1995). *Violence Against Women: Estimates from the Redesigned Survey, August 1995.* NCJ-15438. Special Report. Washington, DC: Government Printing Office.

TAZWELL COUNTY FIRE DEPARTMENT
WORKPLACE VIOLENCE PREVENTION PROGRAM
MAY 12, 1999

The Tazwell County Fire Department is concerned and committed to our employees' safety and health. We refuse to tolerate violence in the workplace and will make every effort to prevent violent incidents from occurring by implementing a Workplace Violence Prevention Program (WVPP). We will provide adequate authority and budgetary resources to responsible parties so that our goals and responsibilities can be met.

All managers and supervisors are responsible for implementing and maintaining our WVPP. We encourage employee participation in designing and implementing our program. We require prompt and accurate reporting of all violent incidents whether or not physical injury has occurred. We will not discriminate against victims of workplace violence.

A copy of this Policy Statement and our WVPP is readily available to all employees from each manager and supervisor.

Our program ensures that all employees, including supervisors and managers, adhere to work practices that are designed to make the workplace more secure, and do not engage in verbal threats or physical actions which create a security hazard for others in the workplace.

All employees, including managers and supervisors, are responsible for using safe work practices, for following all directives, policies and procedures, and for assisting in maintaining a safe and secure work environment.

The management of our establishment is responsible for ensuring that all safety and health policies and procedures involving workplace security are clearly communicated and understood by all employees. Managers and supervisors are expected to enforce the rules fairly and uniformly.

Our Program will be reviewed and updated annually.

PART 1: THE THREAT ASSESSMENT TEAM

A Threat Assessment Team will be established and part of their duties will be to assess the vulnerability to workplace violence at our establishment and reach agreement on preventive actions to be taken. They will be responsible for auditing our overall Workplace Violence Program.

The Threat Assessment Team will consist of:

Name:	Title:	Phone:
John Smith	Fire Chief	555-1212
Jane Doe	Deputy Fire Chief	555-1234
Frank Kras	Chief of EMS Oper.	555-1233
James Brown	Safety Officer	555-1456
Josh Vines	Training Division	555-1567
Tom Jones	Legal Counsel	555-1678
Sally Field	Personnel	555-1789

The team will develop employee training programs in violence prevention and plan for responding to acts of violence. They will communicate this plan internally to all employees.

The Threat Assessment Team will begin its work by reviewing previous incidents of violence at our workplace. They will analyze and review existing records identifying patterns that may indicate causes and severity of assault incidents and identify changes necessary to correct these hazards. These records include, but are not limited to, OSHA 200 logs, past incident reports, medical records, insurance records, Workers' Compensation records, police reports, accident investigations, training records, grievances, minutes of meetings, etc. The team will communicate with similar local businesses and trade associates concerning their experiences with workplace violence.

Additionally, they will inspect the workplace and evaluate the work tasks of all employees to determine the presence of hazards, conditions, operations, and other situations which might place our workers at risk of occupational assault incidents. Employees will be surveyed to identify the potential for violent incidents and to identify or confirm the need for improved security measures. These surveys shall be reviewed, updated, and distributed as needed or at least once within a two year period.

Periodic inspections to identify and evaluate workplace security hazards and threats of workplace violence will be performed by the following representatives of the Assessment Team, in the following areas of our workplace:

Representative: __John Smith__   Area: __General Office Areas__

Representative: __Frank Kras__   Area: __Apparatus Room and Shops__

Representative: __Jane Doe__   Area: __Parking Lots__

Periodic inspections will be performed according to the following schedule:

__First Monday of Every Month__

Frequency (Daily, weekly, monthly, etc.)

PART 2: HAZARD ASSESSMENT

On ___(date)___, the Threat Assessment Team completed the hazard assessment. This consisted of a records review, inspection of the worksite, and employee survey.

A. Records Review—The Threat Assessment Team reviewed the following records:

- __X__ OSHA 200 logs for the last three years

- __X__ Incident reports

- __X__ Records of or information compiled for recording of assault incidents or near assault incidents

- __X__ Insurance records

- _____ Police reports

- _____ Accident investigations

- _____ Training records

- __X__ Grievances

- __X__ Other relevant records or information: __Workers' Compensation records__

From these records, we have identified the following issues that need to be addressed:

- Paramedics have been assaulted by irate patients;
- Office/civilian staff have been assaulted while traveling alone;
- There have been several incidents of assault and harassment among employees.

PART 3: WORKPLACE SECURITY ANALYSIS

A. Inspection—The Threat Assessment Team inspected the workplace on ———(date)———.

From this inspection the following issues have been identified:

- Access to the station, including offices, is not controlled, and it is not limited to any of the offices open to the general public. There have been problems with non-employees entering firefighters' living areas;
- Doors to the restrooms are not kept locked;
- Lighting in the parking lot is inadequate.

B. Review of Tasks—The Threat Assessment Team also reviewed the work tasks of our employees to determine the presence of hazards, conditions, operations and situations which might place workers at risk of occupational assault incidents. The following factors were considered:

- Exchange of money with the public
- Working alone or in small numbers at odd hours
- Working late at night or early in the morning hours
- Providing services in a high crime area
- Safeguarding valuable property or possessions
- Working in community settings
- Staffing levels

From this analysis, the following issues have been identified:

- Employees in office area accept payments from EMS patient billing;
- There are several civilian employees who work very late hours or come in very early in the morning in the office and fire prevention bureau.

PART 4: WORKPLACE SURVEY

Under the direction of the Threat Assessment Team, we distributed a survey among all of our employees to identify any additional issues that were not noted in the initial stages of the hazard assessment. From that survey, the following issues have been identified:

- Employees who work in the field have experienced threats of and acts of violence on several occasions, and there have been several near miss incidents. Employees noted that they were unsure of how to handle the situation and that they are often afraid to travel by themselves to areas they perceive are dangerous;
- Employees who work directly with the public in the office have also experienced threats, both verbal and physical, from some of the clients.

PART 5: WORKPLACE HAZARD CONTROL AND PREVENTION

In order to reduce the risk of workplace violence, the following measures have been recommended:

Engineering Controls and Building and Work Area Design

- Employees who have public contact in the station will have their work areas designed to ensure that they are protected from possible threats from their clients.
- Changes to be completed as soon as possible include:
  - Arranging desks and chairs to prevent entrapment of the employees;
  - Removing items from the top of desks, such as scissors, staplers, etc., that can be used as a weapon;
  - Installing panic buttons to assist employees when clients threaten them. One's foot can activate the buttons. The signal will be transmitted to a supervisor's desk, as well as the security desk, which is always staffed.

Management has instituted the following as a result of the workplace security inspection and recommendations made by the Threat Assessment Team:

- Installation of plexiglass payment window for employees who handle money and need to take payments from clients (number of employees who take money will be strictly limited);
- Adequate lighting systems installed for indoor building areas as well as areas around the outside of the facility and in the parking areas. The lighting systems will be maintained on a regular basis to ensure safety to all employees;
- Locks have been installed on restroom doors and keys given to each department. Restroom doors are to be kept locked at all times. Supervisors will ensure that the keys are returned to ensure continued security for employees in their areas.
- Installation of panic buttons in employees work areas.
- Memorandum to all employees requesting that they remove any items from their desks that can be used as a weapon, such as scissors, staplers, etc.

These changes were completed by ____(date)____.

Policies and Procedures developed as a result of the Threat Assessment Team recommendations:

- Employees who are required to work in the field and who feel that the situation is unsafe should communicate their concerns to the police.
- Employees who work in the field will report to their supervisor periodically throughout the day. They will be provided with a personal beeper or cellular phone, which will allow them to contact assistance should an incident occur.
- Access to the building will be controlled. All civilian employees and sworn employees have been given a name badge, which is to be worn at all times. If employees come in early, or are working past 7:30 p.m., they must enter and exit through the main entrance.
- Visitors will be required to sign in at the front desk. All clients must enter through the main entrance to gain access.

PART 6: TRAINING AND EDUCATION

Training for all employees, including managers and supervisors, was given on ____(date)____. This training will be repeated every two years.

Training included:

- A review and definition of workplace violence;
- A full explanation and full description of our program (all employees were given a copy of this program at orientation);
- Instructions on how to report all incidents, including threats and verbal abuse;
- Methods of recognizing and responding to workplace security hazards;
- Training on how to identify potential workplace security hazards (such as no lights in parking lot while leaving late at night, unknown person loitering outside the building, etc.)
- Review of measures that have been instituted in this organization to prevent workplace violence including:
  - Use of security equipment and procedures;
  - How to attempt to diffuse hostile or threatening situations;
  - How to summon assistance in case of an emergency or hostage situation;
  - Post-incident procedures, including medical followup and the availability of counseling and referral.

Additional specialized training was given to:

- EMS providers in the field;
- Office employees who handle money with clients;
- Employees who work after hours or come in early.

Specialized training included:

- **Personal safety;**
- **Self-defense/aggression management;**
- **Importance of the buddy system;**
- **Recognizing unsafe situations and how to handle them during off-hours.**

This training was conducted by in-house staff, with assistance from the local police department on _____(date)_____ and will be repeated every two years.

At the end of each training session, employees are asked to evaluate the session and make suggestions on how to improve the training.

All training records are filed with _____**the Human Resource/Personnel Department**_____.

Workplace Violence Prevention training will be given to new employees as part of their orientation.

A general review of this program will be conducted every two years. Our training program will be updated to reflect changes in our Workplace Violence Prevention Program.

PART 7: INCIDENT REPORTING AND INVESTIGATION

All incidents must be reported within 8 hours. An "Incident Report Form" will be completed for all incidents. One copy will be forwarded to the Threat Assessment Team for their review and a copy will be filed with _____**the Human Resource/Personnel Department**_____.

The Threat Assessment Team will evaluate each incident. The team will discuss the causes of the incident and will make recommendations on how to revise the program to prevent similar incidents from occurring. All revisions of the program will be put into writing and made available to all employees.

PART 8: RECORDKEEPING

We will maintain an accurate record of all workplace violence incidents. All incident report forms will be kept for a minimum of 7 years, or for the time specified in the Statute of Limitations for our local jurisdiction.

Any injury which requires more than first aid, is a lost-time injury, requires modified duty, or causes loss of consciousness, will be recorded on the OSHA 200 log. Doctor's reports and supervisors' reports will be kept of each recorded incident, if applicable.

Incidents of abuse, verbal attack, or aggressive behavior, which may be threatening to the employee, but not resulting in injury, will be recorded. The Threat Assessment Team will evaluate these records on a regular basis.

Minutes of the Threat Assessment Team meetings shall be kept for 3 years. Records of training program contents, and the sign-in sheets of all attendees, shall be kept for 5 years. Qualifications of the trainers shall be maintained along with the training records.

TAZWELL COUNTY FIRE DEPARTMENT

DEPARTMENT: ADMINISTRATION   **POLICY NUMBER:**

**TITLE: WORKPLACE VIOLENCE PREVENTION
         PLAN AND ZERO TOLERANCE PLAN**

I. PURPOSE

The Workplace Violence Prevention Plan is used to identify violence prone areas and operations in the TAZWELL COUNTY FIRE DEPARTMENT and the measures needed to reduce the potential for violence to occur as much as possible.

II. SCOPE

This policy affects all TAZWELL COUNTY FIRE DEPARTMENT facilities and personnel.

III. PRACTICE

The TAZWELL COUNTY FIRE DEPARTMENT strives to provide a safe environment for everyone who is present in or on the property, or with whom department personnel interact or have contact with. This Workplace Violence Prevention Plan has been developed and is part of the department's Risk Management Program.

1. Responsibilities

   a. In support of the safety of staff, visitors, and those we serve, TAZWELL COUNTY FIRE DEPARTMENT has taken a "Zero-Tolerance" stance in dealing with incidents of violence or threats of violence, and will take appropriate action against any staff member who commits an act of violence/threat. Administration will also ensure the resources and training needed to accomplish this plan are allocated, as deemed necessary.

   b. Staff members are responsible for and are expected to report any and all threats/acts of violence to their supervisor or security. At no time will any reprisal be made against any staff member who reports violent behavior.

   c. Staff are also responsible for following the recommendations made for their safety to assist in reducing the chances of their being the victim of a violent act.

   d. The Safety Committee at each facility has the overall operational responsibility for the safety program, which includes the implementation of this plan.

2. Risk Assessments—Risk Assessments on the potential for violence will be made concurrently with the safety audits. Recommendations for corrective action will be made to the Safety Officer or training Officer of the department. Results will also be reported to the Safety Committee on an as needed basis.

3. Education—The Safety Committee will be responsible for developing and implementing programs to educate all employees of the facility on workplace violence. Staff will receive initial training during New Employee Orientation and refresher training annually.

4. Reporting—All incidents of violence or threats of violence will be reported to the Safety Committee, whether an emergency response is needed or not. These reports will allow the safety committee to trend the activity and see if additional training or other measures are needed to protect personnel in the facility.

5. Employee Background Checks—Staff hired or job applicants being offered positions will receive criminal background checks in accordance with established policies. All regulated and licensed staff will also have a check conducted of their professional licenses. Any information received which reveals past violent behavior may result in the employee/applicant being terminated or not considered for employment.

IV. APPROVAL

This policy is issued by the TAZWELL COUNTY FIRE DEPARTMENT.

Violence in Hospitals

When Violence Comes in the Door . . .

"Sonny" Schultz was well known to local police. At 22 years old, he had been running drug deliveries and cash returns for a local gang since he was 13. Often stopped by police on suspicion, he had never been caught carrying anything, but his activities were no secret to anyone. Today was going to be no exception. Sonny was going to carry one of his biggest deliveries ever.

In the ER, Dr. Chip Morgan was enjoying a surprisingly quiet day. Aside from the routine earaches and sore throats, the day had been extremely slow by trauma center standards. Dr. Morgan was starting back toward the lounge to refill his coffee when he heard the radio used by the ambulances to call in patient transports.

Memorial Hospital from Ambulance 2154 . . . we have a gunshot victim. Our patient is a male, approximately 20 years of age. He has an entrance wound under the left eye, with no visible exit wound. Size weapon is unknown. He is pulseless and the monitor shows asystole. We are performing CPR. One large-bore IV has been established and the patient has been intubated. We are transporting with an ETA of three minutes. . . ."

At the emergency room entrance, Security Officer Jim Madden listened to the scanner, monitoring the call. Knowing the district the ambulance was from, he was certain he would soon have his hands full. The district was "the hood" . . . the portion of the city known for poverty, crime, prostitution, drug dealing, and gang activity. Whenever a violent crime victim was brought in from the hood, dozens of visitors usually followed. Some were legitimate family members, while others had their own agendas. Regardless, he thought, the silence of the ER waiting area would soon be changing.

Radio, 2154 is at Memorial Hospital.

With that radio call, the ER sprang into action. The patient was wheeled in and placed in the trauma room. The trauma team went into precise movements, having been through the routine hundreds if not thousands of times before. And this episode soon ended like many others before it. Only this time, it was Sonny Schultz dead on an ER table . . . shot in retaliation by a rival gang member. As was standard in all violent crimes, the clothing that he had been wearing was secured in a plastic bag to provide to the police . . . no doubt valuable evidence.

In the waiting room, a crowd of about 25 had gathered. Security tried to control the visitors and keep them in one area, but their attempts seemed futile. Soon, Dr. Morgan walked into the waiting area and tried to identify family members. It's useless, he thought . . . everybody is family. Rather than continue attempting to isolate the immediate family, Dr. Morgan instead informed the entire waiting room of the unfortunate outcome.

The response was overwhelming. While an older woman, who was identified as his mother, screamed and then fainted, four young males stormed the ER doors, trying to push past security and a handful of hospital employees. A nurse in the ER screamed while another dialed 911: "We have a riot in the ER at Memorial Hospital!" the panicked voice screamed. The pile soon ended up on the floor, and Jim Madden felt something cold and painful in his abdomen. At first he was stunned, and then he realized he had been stabbed in the brawl. As police arrived, Jim grabbed fellow officer Kurt Vickery by the arm. "Help me, Kurt . . . I'm hurt. . . ."

• • • • • • • • • •

Jim Madden's injuries turned out to be minor. This scenario, based on an actual event, played out for one reason. The victim's pockets were filled with packets of crack cocaine—over $2,000 worth in street value. When he died in the ER, the gang he was running for was at risk of losing their product to the custody of the police. In the absence of the police, they took a chance and tried to overpower the staff. Their actions weren't driven by grief over the loss of a friend or loved one; rather they were driven by the need to recover their investment in illegal drugs and to avoid being accountable to "higher authorities" on the street.

Could this incident have been avoided? In a word: absolutely. First, the hospital staff should have realized that, faced with the large number of visitors gathering, a problem was imminent. Second, arrangements should have been made to inform the immediate family of the victim's death in a more private area, away from outsiders. Third, local police should have been notified immediately when the victim arrived in the ER, in anticipation of a potential problem. Certainly, if the ER staff identified what they suspected might be illegal drugs in the victim's clothing, the police should have been called and no further information communicated to family and friends until the police arrived.

Preparing emergency service providers to deal with *potential* problems is as critical as preparing them to deal with actual problems. We drill to be prepared for mass casualty incidents, hazardous material incidents, major fires, and other critical incidents, but how often do we drill to deal with civil disturbances, violent outbreaks, or aggressive behavior?

Like all other providers, hospitals must assess their risks and plan based on that assessment. Beyond fulfilling the regulatory requirements of agencies such as Health Care Finance Administration (HCFA), Joint Commission on the Accreditation of Healthcare Organizations (JCAHO), and state and local agencies, there is a greater reason for hospitals to prepare: *to survive.*

Introduction

The issue of violence in hospitals is not new. Throughout time, hospitals have had to deal with violent behavior at the hands of patients, visitors, and, in some cases, employees. More recently, however, in a society that seems to tolerate violence as an acceptable behavior, the issue of violence against healthcare workers has gained national attention. The Occupational Safety and Health Administration (OSHA) estimates that each year over 1,500,000 service workers are injured nationally. The majority of these are healthcare workers, injured at the hands of patients, family members, and co-workers. This statistic should be a serious concern to healthcare workers and administrators nationally.

As healthcare providers deal with the issue of violence in the workplace, the types of violence can generally be broken down into six categories:

1. Patient against employee
2. Visitor against employee
3. Patient against patient
4. Visitor against patient
5. Employee against employee
6. Violence occurring at outside locations that extends into the hospital or clinic

Each of these types presents unique situations and challenges to the healthcare provider.

Patient Against Employee

Violence against healthcare providers at the hands of patients is one of the most common forms of violence in healthcare. Patients become violent for a number of reasons, including the following:

- Underlying medical conditions
- Underlying psychiatric conditions
- The loss of autonomy that results from hospitalization
- Misperceptions by patients and families in the delivery of health services resulting in frustration, temper, and in some cases, rage
- Reactions to medication or withdrawal from medication
- Abuse of alcohol or drugs

These are but a few of the reasons that patients become violent during hospitalization or treatment, including in the prehospital setting. The healthcare provider must be aware of these underlying causes and be prepared to deal with potential violence prior to approaching a patient.

The healthcare provider's right to defend him- or herself is perceived much differently when dealing with a patient. In most states, laws regarding the use of force allow an individual the right to use a reasonable level of force to protect him- or herself from injury or death. However, a healthcare provider dealing with an aggressive patient may be held to a different standard.

The following two scenarios illustrate hypothetical situations, but they should give you a better understanding of the difference in standards.

Case Scenario 1
You are at the local grocery store. As you leave the grocery store to go to your car, an individual approaches you and begins asking you for money. You make attempts to ignore the individual; however, he persists. No weapon is displayed, and there is no suggestion of violence on the part of the individual. Instead, he continues to repeatedly ask you for a handout. Despite your continued efforts to ignore the individual, he refuses to take no for an answer. As you continue to walk to your car, the individual realizes that you are ignoring him and grabs your arm.

While the laws vary from state to state, it can easily be perceived that the individual made an aggressive act against you. Depending on the total circumstances, you may be justified using some reasonable degree of force to escape the grasp of the individual. Certainly, when the individual grabbed you, you had every right to fear for your safety.

In a healthcare environment, the same cannot be said, although similar circumstances will certainly present. In a day and age when every patient seems to have their own perception of how healthcare should be delivered, it is not uncommon for patients to grab healthcare providers by the arm or by the hand, not necessarily with the intention of harming anyone but possibly to get their attention.

Case Scenario 2

An emergency department nurse is having a very difficult night, handling multiple victims from a motor vehicle accident. All of the victims are from the same vehicle, and all are heavily intoxicated. Injuries range from the "walking wounded" to more serious problems, including one occupant who has a chest tube in place. One particular individual, the driver, has sustained only minor injuries but is causing constant interruptions. Clearly, even in a state of intoxication, the driver is worried about the others. He is constantly calling the nurse, and when she doesn't respond because her attention is required for more injured occupants, he becomes profane with her. She repeatedly asks him to quiet down. As she walks by his bed to get a piece of equipment, he reaches out and grabs her wrist in a very tight hold and refuses to let go. As he holds her wrist, he says, "I was calling you . . . do I have to show you what happens when people ignore me? . . ."

Unlike the example in the grocery store parking lot, if a patient makes physical contact in an attempt to get the attention of the healthcare provider, the healthcare provider is probably not justified in using physical force against the patient. Certainly, one can appreciate the difficulty a properly trained healthcare provider would have convincing a judge and jury that he or she was justified in pushing or striking a patient, regardless of the actions taken by the patient.

Other situations may present circumstances that allow the healthcare provider to use a different degree of force. Mental health units have proven this theory. With adequate staffing, the degree of force considered necessary to deal with the aggressive acts of a patient is limited to those that are necessary to gain control of the patient. The same, however, cannot be said when staffing patterns or individual circumstances result in an unreasonable risk to the healthcare worker.

Take the case of the mental health worker on the midnight shift. She has eleven patients on the unit, and, as is typical for staffing on nights, there may be only two or three employees working on the floor. During the course of the night, she finds herself trapped in the hallway, cornered by a male patient who is known to be violent or aggressive at times. The patient begins to make threatening and suggestive comments, leading the employee to believe that her safety and well-being are in jeopardy. She has no available method to call for help other than to scream, which she hesitates doing for fear of upsetting other patients on the unit. Is she justified in using force to temporarily disable the aggressive patient? Is she putting herself in even greater jeopardy?

Unfortunately, the answer can't be given in a simple yes or no statement. Again, laws in the respective jurisdictions vary, and it is up to the healthcare professional to know and understand the laws regarding this and other use-of-force situations in healthcare settings.

From a healthcare risk management perspective, it is the responsibility of organization management to perform a comprehensive risk assessment. The assessment, if conducted properly, should identify potential areas for violence in the organization. The assessment should be used by management to take appropriate remedial steps, thereby reducing the likelihood of a violent act against an employee.

Visitor Against Employee

It should seem absurd in our society that a visitor would take aggressive actions against a healthcare provider. For the purpose of this text, the term *visitor* is used in the broadest sense. Visitors include not only family members of patients but also others who may be in the facility for purposes other than employment or treatment. In addition to patient family members, the term visitor can include vendors, distributors, repair personnel, delivery personnel, students, and others not directly affiliated with the hospital.

Violence at the hands of visitors is much different from violence at the hands of patients. Again, underlying cause becomes a question. Oftentimes, healthcare providers focus on the medical, physical, and emotional needs of the patient but fail to address the emotional needs of the patient's family. As a result, family members are unintentionally made to feel like outsiders in the situation. The resulting stress is certainly understandable. Healthcare providers must be sensitive to the emotional needs of the family as well as those of the patient. As much as possible, unless the patient indicates otherwise, the family should be kept informed of changes in the patient's condition and treatment plan. Often, the frustration felt by family members during a time of medical crisis results in increased stress levels. If they are already under extreme stress, this frustration many times leads to violent outbursts. Effective communication remains one of the best tools for prevention.

Another type of violence by visitors against employees, which will be discussed in much greater detail later in this chapter, involves domestic violence. Many of us tend to leave our domestic problems at home when we go to work and deal with them only when we return home. In some cases, however, the problems seem to find their way from home to the workplace. Such was the case in one Midwest hospital recently when a nurse was severely injured at the hands of her husband, who had just been served divorce papers he did not expect. The shock that he felt quickly turned to rage. He then drove to the hospital, found his wife, and became physically violent with her. He was stopped only when hospital security officers arrived to restrain and detain him for the local police.

Seldom do we think of violence in hospitals or in healthcare facilities at the hands of spouses, significant others, or other outsiders. Yet healthcare professionals must always be aware of the increasing risk of violence against them at the hands of others from outside of the organization. Also, they must be prepared to deal with these situations as they present themselves.

Patient Against Patient

Violent actions by patients against one another is an equally growing concern in the healthcare field. This becomes especially true in long-term care facilities, where patients may not be mentally cognizant of the appropriateness of their behavior. As a result, they are unable to appreciate the inappropriateness of violence, and when they feel threatened, will spontaneously resort to violence to protect themselves.

In one recent incident, two nursing home residents were involved. The first resident, an 89-year-old female was sitting alone and unattended in a dining area of the home. Another resident, who was able to move freely about the facility in a wheelchair, entered the dining hall. The first resident, who was already in the dining hall and who lived with a diagnosis of organic brain syndrome, did not want the second resident present. The first resident impolitely told the second resident to leave, which the second resident refused to do. The first resident then proceeded to take a broom that was in the dining hall and beat the wheelchair bound resident with the broomstick. The resident in the wheelchair was critically injured, suffering multiple fractures, bruises, and abrasions. She required hospitalization, surgical intervention, and extensive rehabilitation therapy. Needless to say, the nursing home suffered multiple losses as a result of this incident. The subsequent litigation was unpleasant and portrayed a very poor public image of the nursing home, which was otherwise well respected in the community.

Hospitals are not immune to acts of violence between patients either. Being hospitalized is a stressful time. This is true not only in critical cases in which life-threatening conditions exist but also in cases in which the patient will be disabled for a period of time before full recovery.

Any time a person is hospitalized, they are taken out of their normal lifestyle, removed from their normal environment, put into an environment in which they are perceived as knowing nothing, forced onto schedules that they may or may not appreciate, and required to submit to care they may not appreciate. Anyone who has been hospitalized knows that generally the patient is exposed to repeated episodes of unpleasantness. And that doesn't even include the food they are forced to eat. It is no wonder the stress levels go up.

Patients are placed in a room that is in most cases smaller than the average hotel room and forced to share the room as well as their privacy, their medical conditions, and their treatment plans with a complete stranger. Since many hospitals don't even consider the chances of personal bias on the basis of race, religion, ethnicity, and other factors, it is no wonder that the risk of patients becoming agitated to the point of violence against each other increases.

While the healthcare professional may not be able to change the system in which they work, they can protect themselves by being aware of the hazards and by being prepared to deal with them. Participation in training programs, presented by qualified instructors, remains one of the most reliable tools available.

Visitor Against Patient

We have established that periods of hospitalization are extremely stressful on patients and their families. Acts of violence against patients at the hands of visitors does occur. In one West Coast case a number of years ago, a young male visitor was arrested at the hospital after striking his wife, who was hospitalized and bedridden. The individual, allegedly intoxicated at the time, was apparently having trouble being "father and mother" to the couple's young children, while "mom" lay hospitalized. Seemingly, out of frustration, the individual released his anger on his wife, ultimately striking her as he accused her of neglecting their family.

Incidents of violence against patients at the hands of visitors can destroy a hospital, not only because of the litigation that will likely ensue but also because of the community's loss of trust. Who wants to be admitted to a hospital where violence has occurred?

Hospital security professionals often make a comparison between hotels and hospitals. Both have similarities in that they provide lodging, meals, gift shops, parking areas, guest services, and other commonalties and amenities. The same experts are quick to point out, however, the one significant difference between a hotel and a hospital: in a hotel room you get a lock on your door; in a hospital anybody can enter your room at anytime.

Hospitals have an obligation to provide a safe environment for the patient when the patient is in their care. If the hospital performs a comprehensive risk assessment, patient safety and security will be one of the paramount areas of concern. The hospital must take reasonable steps to ensure the personal safety and security of every patient in the hospital. While not common occurrences, incidents such as sexual assaults, infant abductions, and acts of battery have been reported in hospitals nationwide.

Employee Against Employee

In this book, we will spend considerable time looking at the OSHA workplace violence prevention guidelines and other related standards. Regardless of which one is followed, all standards or guidelines addressing the issue of workplace violence have significant commonalties. One of the most significant is the requirement for a zero tolerance policy on employee violence in the workplace.

Whenever an employee arrives at work, they need to feel safe, and they deserve to feel safe. Their environment should be free from threats, violence, harassment, and other security hazards. They should be allowed to perform their duties in a professional manner and environment. No employee should have to work in an environment where they fear for their safety, are subjected to harassment, or have to face confrontation at the hands of other employees.

Acts of violence between employees don't "just happen." Every act of violence, no matter how slight or how significant, starts with one person as the aggressor. When acts of violence occur in the workplace, the institution cannot downplay the severity of the incident. Regardless of the outcome in terms of personal injuries to employees, the institution has an obligation to investigate the incident and to take appropriate remedial action, up to and including possible termination of the involved employees.

It must also be reemphasized that acts of violence are not necessarily limited to physical violence. Under laws affecting the workplace, acts of violence also include verbal threats, verbal abuse (such as name-calling and impolite threats), the intimidating presence of weapons, or harassment in any of its various forms. If any of these conditions are present, the employer has an obligation to address the issue and to take whatever corrective action is required to reconcile the situation.

Finally, some employers have gone as far as signing criminal charges against employees in addition to terminating their employment. While circumstances surrounding the incident will dictate the consequences, such actions on the part of the employer certainly send a strong signal to the employees that any form of violence in the workplace will not be tolerated.

Community Violence

Any time an act of violence occurs in a community, resulting in an injured patient being transported to the hospital, there is significant risk that the cause of the violence may also continue into the hospital. This is especially true in communities with high incidents of violent crime or in hospitals that have a high frequency of trauma victims.

One example involves a suburban hospital, in which an adult male came into the ER with a female patient who had obviously been badly beaten. The male identified himself as a family member of the victim and stated to the emergency room nurses that she came home in this condition. While the patient was taken into another room for treatment, the male was asked to wait in the outer waiting room, along with families of other patients in the ER at the time.

Once in the treatment room, the patient told the nursing personnel that the individual had been holding her against her will and had beaten and repeatedly sexually assaulted her. He had only brought her to the hospital when she lost consciousness during one of the beatings. Nursing personnel quickly notified hospital security, who contacted the local police. Approaching the individual in the waiting room was out of the question due to the risk of injury or harm to other visitors in the room. An alert security officer was able to evacuate all visitors quietly and effectively until the offender was the only person left in the waiting room. Once this was the case, the police entered and took the individual into custody without incident.

Had the security officer in this case not handled the situation the way he did, the outcome could have been catastrophic. The offender in this case could very easily have grabbed another visitor and created a hostage situation. If he was armed, he may very easily have been able to draw a weapon and use it against others present at the time. Although the actions of this professional hospital security officer resulted in a safe outcome in this incident, the case also illustrates how easily outside acts of violence can escalate from the community into the hospital.

Prehospital providers, as well as emergency department and trauma center personnel, must remain acutely aware of this risk and be prepared to deal with it. Prehospital providers often find themselves in situations in which they have a victim and an offender present and no police assistance on the scene. These providers must be aware of the great danger they face in such a situation and must be prepared to deal with their own self-protection as well as the protection of the patient and bystanders at the scene.

In cases in which prehospital providers are responding to the scene of an act of violence, they are well-advised to ascertain if police are on the scene before entering. If police are not physically present at the scene, prehospital providers should then stage at a proximal location until police arrive and it is determined that the scene is safe for them to enter. Again, however, providers must check local laws regarding the duty to act. Specifically, prehospital providers will want to determine if it is legally permissible to stage until the scene has been secured, or if poorly written state laws require them to proceed into the scene under a duty to act without regard for their own safety. In most states, prehospital providers would not be expected to enter a violent scene that is unsafe. However, to be safe, these providers are well-advised to inquire with legal council for an opinion.

Domestic Violence

In addition to workplace violence, domestic violence is a growing crisis in the United States. Many states have now passed legislation requiring the arrest of any individual committing an act of domestic violence, regardless of circumstances. In the past, the victim of domestic violence would have to sign a criminal complaint before law enforcement officials could arrest the offender. In many states, this is no longer true, and when an act of domestic violence occurs, police are required to arrest the offender, regardless of the wishes of the victim.

It cannot be overlooked that domestic violence situations are one of the leading causes of injury and death to police officers. When the officers are called to the scene, they find themselves in the middle of what is often a violent incident between husband/wife, boyfriend/girlfriend, or some other relationship gone bad. In some cases, when police attempt to arrest the offender, the tide suddenly turns, and the "victim" then turns on the police officer.

Although this book is not meant to deal with aggression management tactics for law enforcement, the prehospital provider must always be aware of the risk that he or she is placed in when responding to a domestic violence call for help. Like the police, the prehospital provider will be seen as an authority figure, and when medical treatment is necessary they become the ones who are taking the victim out of the home or another environment. Many prehospital providers and paramedics have been injured while attempting to take a victim of domestic violence out of a residence. Some have been injured when trying to assist police officers when others present started to aggress against the police.

Anyone who believes that a hospital (or the sanctity of an ambulance) is immune from incidents of domestic violence is sadly mistaken. Incidents of domestic violence have occurred in hospitals, clinics, nursing homes, and even in the back of ambulances.

In cases of domestic violence involving employees, it is rare that the first act of violence occurs at work. In most cases, an employee that finds himself or herself the victim of a domestic violence incident at work is probably already living in a violent environment. To protect employees, the employer is well advised to encourage them to discretely report their involvement in an abusive relationship or when there is a risk for domestic violence in the workplace.

While the employer has an obligation to be discreet in protecting the employee's dignity and right to privacy, the employer also has the responsibility to take appropriate action to ensure that the other individual is not afforded the opportunity to enter the facility to commit an act of violence.

For example, a nurse reports to her supervisor that she and her spouse are having marital trouble. In addition, he has recently become physically abusive with her. She informs the nursing supervisor that she fears for her safety. She continues by stating that he has been threatening her since she filed for divorce three weeks ago. He also told her not to fool herself into thinking she was safe at work.

What are some steps management may take to protect this employee and the other employees, patients, and visitors? First, the nursing supervisor should contact hospital security. If possible, the employee should be asked to provide a photograph of her husband, which can be shared with hospital security personnel. Information on the type of automobile driven by the husband should also be shared. The employee should be provided with a security escort to her vehicle at the end of every shift and should be met by security in the employee parking lot when she reports to work at the start of each shift. These are but a few examples of the kinds of proactive steps that can be taken for the protection of employees in the workplace. Obviously, however, it begins with the employee trusting and confiding in the employer about the situation and its potential for violence.

The same consideration must be given to patients when they are at risk. Studies have shown a common behavior pattern when relationships involve domestic violence. The violent person becomes abusive and later becomes apologetic and remorseful. For a variety of reasons, the victim forgives the offender and stays in the relationship. This pattern continues to cycle, with episodes of abuse followed by apologetic and remorseful episodes. The chronically abusive individual does not limit abusive behaviors to the boundaries of home. Abuse can and does occur anywhere.

If a patient is involved in an abusive relationship, the risk of being abused while in the hospital is as great as the risk would be at home. Hospital personnel must be keenly aware of the increased risk to the safety and well-being of their patients when the patients notify them that they are victims of an abusive relationship. Many healthcare professionals hesitate to ask questions that can provide critical information because they "don't want to pry." Many times, the reluctance to ask questions results from an uncertainty on how to approach the subject. According to Dr. Joseph Danna, project medical director at Provena St. Mary's Hospital in Kankakee, Illinois, "a significantly high number of domestic violence victims are seen in the ED, and the domestic violence issues are never recognized or addressed." Dr. Danna goes on to note that "these professionals are doing a serious injustice to their patients and need to be better educated in techniques of recognizing and dealing with victims of domestic violence."

The message is clear and simple. The patient who is involved in an abusive relationship, whether it is with their spouse, immediate family, significant other, co-workers, or others cannot be considered safe and immune from acts of violence simply because they are hospitalized.

Visitors are one more group that is not immune from domestic violence in the hospital. In one hospital case, a male visitor stopped at the hospital to visit a female co-worker. While he was visiting her, her husband arrived to visit. When the husband found another male in the room visiting his wife, he immediately began accusing the wife of having an affair, and a fight ensued between the husband and the male visitor. Fortunately for the visitor, he was well prepared to defend himself, and the husband ended up on the losing end of the situation. By the same token, the case illustrates how easily incidents of domestic violence can occur against visitors as well as any other class or group of individuals present at any time.

Domestic violence against visitors may be one of the most difficult types of aggressive behavior for the hospital to proactively prepare for, since acts of domestic violence against visitors can occur anywhere in the building. Additionally, seldom does the hospital have the opportunity to provide educational programming for visitors on this issue. As a result, there is no real mechanism available to prepare or prevent domestic violence incidents when visitors are involved as victims. Instead, the hospital is better off to focus their preventive efforts on the education of employees in various methods of response and in obtaining emergency assistance when these incidents do occur.

Gang Violence

The U.S. Department of Justice's Office of Juvenile Justice and Delinquency Prevention National Youth Gang Center completed a survey in December of 1996. According to the survey, law enforcement agencies in all 50 states reported that 664,906 gang members belong to 23,388 gangs. Gang activity is not a new phenomenon in the United States, but it continues to be a national concern. Gang culture seems to be growing in every community, small and large. In most instances, gang members have treated the hospital as "off limits," because they recognize the likelihood that they may at some time be treated at the hospital. In other cases, the hospital is treated with no more reverence than any other location. Hospital employees, including nursing, security, and administration, need to know the mind-set of local gangs toward their hospital and be prepared in advance to deal with the unique situations gangs present.

In many cases, the gang member patient is not the problem. Like many other patients, the gang member may appreciate the care and attention that he or she receives. At the same time, fellow gang members may not wish to conform to hospital rules and regulations regarding visitors and instead attempt to intimidate staff, other patients, and visitors.

One of the most effective tools for dealing with gang problems is a strong relationship with local law enforcement agencies. Many times, these agencies are knowledgeable about the gangs in their communities. Some even know individual gang members and the role each plays in the gang.

The presence of law enforcement officers may also be beneficial in maintaining a state of calm in the facility. While few hospitals go to the extreme of hiring police officers to be present in the hospital, having local police immediately available is a strong tool of prevention.

In one community heavily plagued with gang activity and associated drug dealing, the local police have entered into an agreement with the hospital designed to reduce or eliminate the risk of gang activity when gang members are being treated. Under the agreement, whenever an act of violence occurs in the community involving a known or suspected gang member or gang location, a police officer is automatically dispatched to the hospital emergency department. As a result, police are physically present in the emergency department, often before the injured party arrives. The presence of the uniformed police, in addition to the hospital uniformed security staff, serves as a deterrent. Upon arrival, other gang members are met at the doors and turned away. As a result, the hospital has seen a 90% reduction in the incidents of gang-related violence in the emergency department or hospital.

Bomb Threats, Riots, and Civil Unrest

Healthcare workers must also be prepared for acts of violence that occur within a community but not necessarily within the boundaries of their own institution. These acts include bomb threats, riots, and civil unrest. Often, prehospital providers are called to the scene of these activities, whether there have been any casualties or not. They need to be prepared to treat the victims of an actual bombing, riot, or civil disturbance—not an easy task for most of us. Responding to violence in each of these situations requires preplanning. Most hospital and prehospital providers participate in emergency preparedness drills. These drills should include response to bombings, riots, and civil disturbances. Like any other type of disaster, the creation of an emergency plan is necessary. Following is a list of guidelines for creating this plan:

- Meet with local police, fire, prehospital, and hospital disaster planning committees.
- Discuss responsibilities of each agency in response to each of the aforementioned disaster types.
- For prehospital providers, determine in advance how victims will be removed from an area where danger may still be present. This may require a police escort, or, in some cases, may require waiting until the danger subsides. It's better to know in advance than to make a critical decision under stressful circumstances.
- Post emergency telephone numbers near telephones and in other easy-to-locate areas.
- Assemble a list of emergency supplies in addition to the ones you already carry.
- Know the limitations of the emergency departments in your response area.
- Know the procedures for bypass of local emergency departments.

Summary

According to a report released on August 24, 1997 by the U.S. Bureau of Justice Statistics, 1.4 million people were treated in hospital emergency rooms for violence-related injuries. Of those, approximately 17% were injured by people they had an intimate relationship with—a spouse, former spouse, boyfriend, girlfriend, or former boyfriend or girlfriend. Sixty percent of the injured were males. In addition, nearly 50% of the victims were injured by someone they knew, while only 23% were injured by strangers. Alarmingly, the report indicated this was four times higher than estimates by the U.S. Bureau of Justice Statistics National Crime Victimization Survey, one of the nation's foremost sources of crime victim data. Of those emergency department reports that indicated a location, 48% occurred in the home.

With over 1.4 million violence-related victims treated in the nation's hospitals, what do you think the odds are that you'll be involved in a violent incident at some point in your career? Despite the odds being stacked against you, you do not have to become a victim. Through proper planning, training, and drilling exercises, you can increase the odds of being able to handle a violent incident, without sacrificing yourself in the process.

References

Occupational Safety and Health Administration (OSHA). (1996). OSHA Workplace Violence Awareness and Prevention Facts and Information. Fact Sheet No. OSHA 96-53. www.osha.gov.

U.S. Department of Justice's Office of Juvenile Justice and Delinquency Prevention National Youth Gang Center. (December 1996). www.usdoj.gov.

U.S. Bureau of Justice Statistics. (August 1997). *Violence Related Injuries Treated in Hospital Emergency Departments*. Washington, DC: Government Printing Office.

The PREVENT® Plan for Violence

"Not Being Prepared Almost Got Us Killed"

"An ounce of prevention is worth a pound of cure." We've all heard that saying many times in our lives but never did it have so much meaning as the day we were called to the scene of a shooting. The dispatcher told us that the complainant stated that there were shots fired and they could hear someone crying for help.

We thought we were well prepared. We arrived at the scene at about 2:30 A.M. We weren't sure if the perpetrator(s) were still present, so we did the right thing and waited for police backup. Although unfortunate, since one of our paramedics was killed in the line of duty while trying to treat a woman who was beaten severely during a domestic incident, it is our policy to wait for the police before entering a crime scene. We didn't have to wait long. The police arrived within one minute of us and planned their entry. Within another minute there were at least five squad cars and nine police officers. One of the officers, obviously the shift supervisor, was directing some of the patrolmen to go around to the back, while others were getting equipment out of the trunks of their cars. They had obviously done this before. Everything seemed to be synchronized. We were impressed. Within another two or three minutes, the police officers were waving at us to come inside. We had a stretcher and jump kit ready and proceeded inside. When we walked through the doors we saw blood everywhere.

There were two victims, a male and a female. The male victim was an obvious "triple zero"—no pulse, no respiration, no blood pressure. His head was partially severed from his body. The female victim was bleeding profusely from the head. Upon examining the female, we discovered she had been cut on the scalp and her hands and arms. Although the type of wound she had caused her to bleed abundantly, it was not all that severe. We began to clean and bandage the wounds, when someone came running in to the apartment shouting, "They're right outside. The guys that did this are right outside." One of the police officers grabbed the guy and handcuffed him. The officer then started questioning the guy about what he knew. After a couple of seconds, the guy calmed down enough to tell the officers that he had seen three teenagers running from the victims' apartment right before the ambulance arrived. The officers all went outside to see if they could locate the alleged offenders.

In the meantime, we were treating the elderly female subject and notified the hospital of the situation. Just as we were ready to transport, a male teenage subject entered the room. To this day nobody knows exactly where he came from. He was holding a huge knife; I think it was a machete. He was covered with blood and shaking so badly he could barely stand. He told us to be quiet or we would get the same thing the "old people got." There were three of us, and we all froze. It was as if time had suddenly stopped. Everything seemed to be going in slow motion. I'm not sure who was more scared, the teenager or us. I must have had twenty-five thoughts go through my mind in a matter of seconds. I thought about shouting but was afraid that would push this kid over the edge. I thought about rushing him and trying to get the machete out of his hand. That's when my thoughts changed to friends and family. I thought about my little girl who was expecting me to wake her up and get her ready for school in the morning. I thought about my wife who always told me she didn't sleep well knowing the kinds of calls I had to go on. I thought about my neighbor who drove over my freshly planted flowers on my driveway this morning. How stupid I was for being so mad. I know he didn't do it on purpose. I even thought about what a great lady I had for my boss. That's when I knew I must be delirious.

After a few minutes the teenage boy told us to take the "old bitch" off the stretcher. We carefully removed the lady to her sofa. The teenage boy then walked over and lay on the stretcher. He said, "cover me up and take me out to the ambulance. After placing the sheet over him, he said, "If you make any false moves or say anything to alert the cops, I'll kill all of you." Again, we complied. As I was pushing the stretcher toward the ambulance, I noticed several police officers searching the area with flashlights. I wanted to shout but was afraid this kid would kill my partners or me. As I reached the ambulance and started to load the stretcher, I once again thought about alerting the police but quickly changed my mind. I loaded the stretcher and got in the back with him. My partners got in front and started to drive away. We got about a half-mile from the scene when the kid told us to stop. He ordered us out of the ambulance. He made us lie down in a ditch and told us we would not get hurt if we complied. The next thing I remember is seeing the ambulance drive away. Shortly afterward, we saw three squad cars go speeding by, and another one stopped to pick us up.

• • • • • • • • • •

As I think about the situation today, I realize how poorly prepared we were for this situation. There were more mistakes made than we can even count. We were just fortunate that none of us were killed. That's the last time I go to any call without being totally prepared, mentally and physically.

Introduction: Being Prepared

Imagine for a moment that you are preparing for a two-week vacation. What are some of the things you would need to do to prepare? If you were driving you would most likely take your vehicle in for a checkup before leaving. The night before you leave, you would likely gas up your vehicle and check all the fluids. You would make sure you have a map to the location you are traveling. You would make hotel arrangements. If you were a really prepared traveler, you would probably even make an itinerary of what you would do each day you are on vacation. If you were flying, you would purchase your tickets and make arrangements for a car rental. These are just a few of the things you would do before leaving. And this doesn't include getting someone to watch your house, water your plants, feed your pets, take in your mail and newspapers, and so on. Most of that is simple common sense. You make all these preparations, and we're talking about a vacation . . . certainly not something considered life threatening.

In prehospital situations, however, you deal with life-threatening circumstances all the time, not only involving your own life but someone else's life as well. How many calls would you respond to without knowing you have the proper medical equipment and supplies to handle any given situation? Think how embarrassing, and life threatening, it would be to arrive at an accident scene without the equipment needed to immobilize a cervical spine injury. Of course this sounds ridiculous. If your department is like most, there is an equipment and supply inventory that must be completed regularly. Even the smallest departments in the country know better than to leave the station without proper equipment. Why? Experience has taught us what equipment is needed on most calls. And it is no different when dealing with aggressive patients.

Experience shows that prehospital providers are finding themselves in increasingly dangerous situations. Although they know they will respond to a dangerous situation or two, or even a thousand during their career, how many actually plan what they will do before violence occurs?

When teaching crime prevention or aggression management, instructors often ask students to stand, look around the room, and point to the person who is most likely to become a victim of violence. In most instances, students will look around the room and point to a person who is either petite or timid looking. Rarely do students point to themselves. Mostly everyone believes that violence only happens to other people. Prehospital providers are no different. They think they will be called to treat someone else who has been involved in a violent incident. They certainly don't think they will be the victim.

In planning for violence, prehospital providers must first realize and understand that they are in a profession in which violence should be anticipated. They must understand that they are vulnerable and are just as likely to become the victim of violence as anyone else. A prehospital provider will encounter all types of violent behaviors, including domestic violence, child abuse, elder abuse, gang violence, sexual assault, and drug-related violence, in addition to criminal activity up to and including homicide. In many cases, the prehospital provider will not know if the person being treated is a victim or the perpetrator of violence. No matter what, the prehospital provider must deliver prompt, professional medical assistance, without bias. This chapter focuses on the many ways prehospital providers can prepare themselves for violence on every call in the same way they prepare to respond to any emergency situation.

The best method for reducing violence is to prevent it from happening in the first place. Easier said than done, of course. However, by being prepared to PREVENT® violence and to take the initiative to train, drill, and practice these methods, the prehospital provider can reduce the likelihood of being victimized by violence. Called the PREVENT® program to help make it easier to learn and remember, much of what is contained in this chapter is basic common sense. For this program to be effective the prehospital provider must learn what each letter in the PREVENT® program stands for, teach the program to others, and implement it in his or her department.

There are four basic steps in the pre-plan phase of the PREVENT® program:

Step 1: Assess Vulnerability

Take responsibility. Do not wait until you become the victim of violence yourself. Conduct an assessment of past incidents. Review injury reports, accident reports, OSHA 200 logs, and other records to determine where your vulnerability lies. Incident trending may give you information such as:

- The location(s) where most violent incidents occur
- The day of week most incidents occur
- The name(s) of patients who have a history of violence
- The time of day most incidents occur
- The number and types of injuries sustained in violent confrontations

If your department is like most, you probably have a preconceived idea of when and where violence occurs. How many of you have heard, or participated in, the following conversation:

ER Nurse: *"Looks like a full moon tonight."*

ER Doctor: *"Why do I always pull a 24 (hour shift) every time there is a full moon?"*

Paramedic: *"Yeah, well the ambulance will be running nonstop tonight too."*

How many times have you discussed how busy it will be on Labor Day, Memorial Day, the 4th of July, Friday and Saturday night, and New Year's Eve? But do you really have the statistics to prove these theories? Few departments actually keep these figures, but this information could be helpful in developing specific work practices and staffing patterns.

For example, your assessment may determine that Sunday nights are busier than Friday and Saturday, but your staffing is lowest on Sunday. A simple change in staffing could make a world of difference when confronting a violent patient. Simple things may provide you with a completely different insight into where your real risks lie.

Step 2: Assess Equipment

When responding to a call, you try to have all equipment necessary to effect quality patient care. But what about personal protective equipment (PPE)? We are talking, of course, about personal protective equipment to protect you from violence. In addition to latex gloves, impervious gowns, face masks, face shields, and eye protection, PPEs for violence should not be an afterthought. Numerous protective devices are available to help reduce the risk for violence. These not only include restraint devices and safety straps, but also the following items.

Closed-Circuit TV (CCTV) Cameras
Once thought to be used only in the retail industry, CCTV is widely and effectively used in business and industry as a deterrent to criminal activity. CCTV cameras are being effectively used in school buses, police cars, and public transportation. Even when a crime does occur, CCTV often successfully records criminal activity and helps authorities to resolve

crime. It has also been successful in civil lawsuits against police departments where the claim of excessive force has been made and to show the condition of the offender (e.g., intoxicated, violent, uncooperative). CCTV could also help you/your department when a combative patient makes a claim that he/she was the model patient.

Personal Alarm Devices

There are many types of personal alarm devices on the market. If you are also a firefighter, as many prehospital providers are, you are probably familiar with the PASS device. This device emits a high-decibel alarm if you run into trouble as well as an automatic alarm feature that activates if you become motionless for a predetermined period of time. These and other types of personal alarms may also be used for prehospital providers who often enter volatile situations and need to call for assistance in a hurry. Depending on your budget and the degree of risk you are routinely exposed to, you may even need a more elaborate system, one that transmits a distress signal not only locally but also to your radio communications center, where dispatchers are able to summon police assistance for you. You should carefully assess the need for these devices and be familiar with the various systems available on the market.

Geographic Locating Devices

Chances are that you never imagined your ambulance being stolen. But think about it, how many times a day do you park your ambulance with the keys in the ignition and the engine running? Obviously your answer will depend in part on the number of calls you make. However, most departments do not have the staff to leave someone with the ambulance at all times, and you don't want to shut off your engine for fear the vehicle may not start at a crucial time when someone's life is in jeopardy. Why are ambulances stolen? In a word: drugs! Many ambulances are "Pharmacies on Wheels." And even if yours is not, how does the thief know? Ambulances are prime targets for theft and should have a geographic locating device installed to expedite rapid recovery. The longer your ambulance is out of service, the longer someone may have to wait for the next one.

Body Armor

Some departments have chosen body armor for their prehospital providers. Body armor has helped save lives. For example, the lives of more than 1,800 police officers have been saved by bullet proof vests (Brierley, 1996). We are not saying every prehospital provider should have a bulletproof vest, but if the department or agency knows they will be providing services in an area known for violent crime, then they should give careful consideration to providing these devices on every ambulance and require their use when circumstances dictate. Also look beyond your primary response area. If you provide mutual aid services, you need to look at the areas you are commonly called into, places where the risk may be greater than in your primary response areas.

Step 3: Assess Vehicle Condition

No matter what type of ambulance, fire apparatus, or other transportation your department uses, it must be well maintained. Before you begin your shift, check to make sure you have a full tank of fuel. Keeping the fuel tank full not only keeps you from running out but can also help keep moisture or condensation from forming in your tank. This moisture can cause a frozen fuel line in the winter or a vapor lock in the summer. Check also your oil, windshield washer fluid, brake fluid, power steering fluid, and proper working equipment such as lights, sirens, horns, and radios. It would also be wise to check the air pressure in each of the tires. A tire with less air than the rest may indicate a slow leak. You need to report the leak so that you do not end up with a flat tire at the worst possible moment. Most of all, have a well-trained, certified mechanic keep your vehicle maintained in accordance with the manufacturer's recommendations. After all, that vehicle may provide your only means of escape. Most all departments include daily vehicular checks as part of an ongoing preventive maintenance program. Make sure yours is comprehensive and complete at the start of each shift. Although it may not be an exciting part of the day, it may be a life-saving one.

Step 4: Assess Yourself

Are you prepared to handle a violent confrontation? As you are driving to the scene of your next call, consider how you would handle a violent patient. What would you do if the patient lunged toward you while you were conducting your initial assessment? What would you do if the patient grabbed your arm while you are trying to start an IV? Better yet, think of the last time your knees were knocking so loudly that you could not hear yourself think. How will you handle a similar situation the next time it occurs? A positive mental attitude is often the simplest way to defuse potentially violent situations. Thinking through the various possibilities in your mind will help you do the right things should such a situation arise.

R = Recognize Dangers

Be alert to your surroundings at all times. Whenever possible, park your ambulance in a well-lit area. You were trained to provide rapid response to medical emergencies but that does not mean you have to put yourself in danger. Remember, you cannot provide medical care if you get yourself hurt or killed. Even an armed police officer does not hurry into a dangerous situation without carefully assessing the surroundings and making sure plenty of assistance is available. Always assess the surroundings before approaching a situation. What are you getting into? If you are responding to the scene of a shooting, stabbing, fight, domestic dispute, or other criminal incident, has the offender been apprehended? Are the police present? Is there a hostile crowd? In some cases, you may have to wait for the police to arrive to escort you to the scene. When you enter a building or residence, always observe at least two routes of exit, and make sure there is a clear path between you and the exits. Pay attention to who is around you at all times. Do not let yourself be distracted. In addition, pay close attention for items in the vicinity that might be used as weapons against you—large ash trays, lamps, tables, chairs, fireplace tools, knives, and guns, to name a few. And do not forget those things you carry that could be used as a weapon against you—hypodermic needles, stethoscopes, blood pressure cuffs, scissors. The list goes on and on. Whenever possible, remove as many of these items from the area as you can. Remember, even a patient who is showing no signs of distress may, for no apparent reason, become violent. Do not become a statistic because you did not take the time to survey your surroundings. In some buildings, you may have to use elevators. If so, always stand away from the doors, wait for the doors to open completely, and look to be sure no one is hiding inside before entering. It would also be wise to make sure that there is an elevator car present when the doors open. Ridiculous as it sounds, many people have died senseless deaths because they stepped into the elevator when the door opened and fell into an open shaft.

E = Evaluate Options

If a violent patient confronts you, what should you do?

Do you retreat and wait for backup?

Many would argue that the only viable option for a prehospital provider is to retreat and wait for backup. After all, you are not the police. You should not be expected to confront a violent patient under any circumstance. However, what if the violent patient has a head injury and is wandering around the scene of an accident? By retreating and waiting for backup, are you endangering the life of the patient even more? Are you responsible if the patient collapses and dies? What if the patient wanders into traffic and gets struck by another vehicle?

Do you engage the patient?

Again, some would say prehospital providers should never fight with a patient. They are neither paid to fight with patients, nor are they trained to fight. They are only there to treat the condition exhibited by the patient. Others, however, believe that prehospital providers should be allowed to use whatever force is necessary to treat the patient. After all, they are only looking out for the best interest of the patient, and isn't that what they are trained to do? Chapter 5 covers this topic in-depth; however, under most circumstances, prehospital providers are only allowed to fight with a patient to protect themselves, the patient, other bystanders, or property.

Are you carrying a portable radio or other communication device?

Most departments have radios in their squads, but do you carry one with you to every call? If your department does not supply a portable radio or cellular phone, think about investing in one yourself. Cellular phones are extremely affordable and may even save your life. They are well worth the investment if you only use them for emergency purposes.

Do you have items or tools available to handle a confrontation?

Earlier in the chapter, several personal protective items were discussed, including closed circuit television, personal alarm devices, body armor, and geographic locating devices. They cannot help you if they are left at the station. Have you checked to make sure you have proper restraint devices?

It may not be possible to answer each of these questions until you are confronted with the issue, but the more you answer now, the better prepared you will be. You must know your department policy; federal, state, and local laws; and the standard operating procedures of your prehospital system. Carefully thought out options are crucial for life safety in the event of a violent confrontation and should always be part of your pre-plan and your response.

V = Value Resources

What resources do you have available? Does the department back you up on service calls? Do you have two-way communications with the fire and/or police department? Is training provided to help prepare you to deal with aggressive or violent behavior? In some agencies, these topics are not addressed because the person who should be addressing them does not believe it will happen in his or her department.

The person who takes this attitude is probably the same person who goes to a fire with no water in the booster tank of the engine because "there are never fires around here anyway."

Always remember that prehospital providers and paramedics have been injured at the hands of violent patients in both small towns and urban areas. Prepare yourself. Make certain the training and equipment needed to protect yourself is available, and make a personal commitment to yourself to train and take advantage of every bit of training and equipment available.

E = Exercise Regularly

Have you ever had to work with a partner who is terribly out of shape? We are talking about someone who is so overweight that they become short-winded just walking across the apparatus room floor or up a flight of stairs. If so, you may have worried about that person's ability to perform when the chips are down. And when the chips are down, it's too late to find out.

Whether your department has a physical conditioning program or not, you need to keep yourself in excellent physical condition. The more physically fit you are, the better prepared you will be to handle yourself in a confrontation. As our society continues to develop its "fitness craze," new gyms and fitness programs are popping up everywhere. Even if you have to drive a distance to get to a gym, it will be well worth the time and effort. Some departments will absorb the cost of physical fitness classes for prehospital providers and firefighters. If yours does, take advantage of this generosity. If it does not, sign yourself up anyway. Because there is so much competition between fitness centers, they can often be inexpensive.

Whenever possible, attend self-defense classes. Many police departments and martial arts studios offer from time to time basic self-defense classes. Take advantage of them. If you really cannot afford to attend a gym or to sign up for self-defense classes, do your own aerobic exercises. It does not cost much to go for a jog or run, ride your bike, or take a swim. Whatever method of exercise you choose, do it for at least 30 minutes a day, every day. Always try to maintain a well-balanced diet, because good nutrition will keep you alert and functioning optimally. It is always advisable to check with your physician before beginning any fitness program.

N = Notify Authorities

Whenever you are aware that a criminal activity has occurred, notify the proper authorities. If you are not sure if something is criminal, let the authorities decide. Whether the victim is you or someone else, you have a duty to report the crime that has occurred. After all, you are a public servant. It is also advisable to prosecute the offender to the full extent of the law. How would you feel if you failed to prosecute or bear witness against a criminal only to find out that he or she has committed the same crime or a worse one against someone else?

Another benefit of reporting is the continued collection of data. Early in this chapter, we talked about analyzing data and using it effectively as a management tool. The more data you have available, the more informed your decisions will be.

T = Train, Train, and Train Some More

The need for ongoing training in the recognition and de-escalation of violent behavior cannot be overemphasized. Additionally, if your vulnerability assessment in the pre-plan phase was conducted properly, you probably discovered hazards associated with specific tasks or locations you previously did not know existed. In this phase, it is time to develop and implement relevant behavioral techniques to minimize the potential for violence. You may question why you should change your behavior when you are trying to help; when you have not done anything wrong. Most would agree with you and empathize with your thought process. However, when is the last time you changed someone else's behavior? It was probably a long time ago, if ever. You can influence someone's behavior, but you cannot change it. Therefore, by modifying your behavior you reduce the risk to yourself, your co-workers, and the patient. A competent training program is but one component in a comprehensive approach to reducing workplace violence. To increase compliance with violence prevention techniques, training should emphasize the appropriate use and maintenance of protective equipment, adherence to safe work practices, and increased knowledge and awareness of the risk of violence.

To find out if you are properly trained, ask yourself the following questions:

1. Do you know your department's policy about the use of force?
2. Do you know how to recognize risk factors that cause or contribute to assaults?
3. Do you know how to recognize warning signs and/or symptoms of escalating behavior that may lead to an assault?
4. Have you or your department developed approaches for preventing, defusing, and responding to volatile situations including techniques for managing your own anger?
5. Do you know the location of all personal protective equipment for violence?
6. Do you know what resources are available to assist you if a violent patient confronts you?

How did you do? Do you always prepare in each of the areas we talked about? If so, you are well on your way to a long, successful career. If not, take these recommendations seriously. They may save your life—you and your family both deserve your safe return after each shift.

Summary

A successful outcome starts with preparedness. As a caregiver, you are vulnerable to violence. Take steps to prepare yourself to deal with the risk and to be ready to face situations when they present.

The PREVENT® plan for preparedness gives you the tools to be ready to respond in a crisis situation. The PREVENT® plan is a simple to use acronym that stands for:

P = Pre-plan for situations so you are ready when they present.

R = Recognize dangers. . .avoid being "blindsided" by a situation.

E = Evaluate your options and choose the option that offers you the most safety and security.

V = Value available resources and take advantage of them.

E = Exercise regularly. Staying in shape may play a key role in saving your life in a crisis situation.

N = Notify authorities whenever you are made aware that a crime has occurred, regardless of the source of the information.

T = Train. Train again. Train some more. You cannot over train in techniques of aggression management and de-escalation.

Nothing can guarantee a successful outcome each and every time. Since circumstances and conditions vary, outcomes can be equally varied. Still, using the tenants of the PREVENT® plan, you will find yourself better prepared and equipped to respond.

Reference

Brierley, B. (1996). Personal communication on February 7, 1996, between B. Brierley of the IACP/Dupont Kevlar Survivors' Club and Lynn Jenkins, Division of Safety Research, National Institute for Occupational Safety and Health, Centers for Disease Control and Prevention, Public Health Service, U.S. Department of Health and Human Services. Cited in *Violence in the Workplace: Risk Factors and Prevention Strategies*. (July 1996). DHHS (NIOSH) Pub. No. 96-100. Cincinnati, OH: National Institute for Occupational Safety and Health. www.cdc.gov/niosh/violrisk.html.

Recognizing Potential Violence: The Aggression Continuum

There Aren't Enough of You to Drag Me Out of Here . . .

"Excuse me sir, but it is 8:50 now. Visiting hours ended at 8:30. You are going to have to leave."

With those words, Esther Montore started a series of events that would not end until a hospital security officer was injured and a concerned husband placed in jail.

"It was the nurse's approach that put me on the defensive, right from the start" according to Bob Fortin, whose wife Judy recently lost a two-year battle with cancer. *"Judy had been battling breast cancer for several years, and we both knew she was losing the battle. She slept better when I was with her, especially on the nights when the pain was more intense. She seemed more relaxed when I would pull a chair next to her bed and just hold her hand until she fell asleep. Most of the nurses were so fantastic, I don't know why this one had to be so Gestapo-like. I had never seen her before, and she better hope I never see her again."*

Esther Montore had been a nurse at the hospital for 17 years, most of them on the med/surg unit. On this particular night, the oncology unit was short two nurses, so the nursing supervisor pulled her from med/surg and reassigned her to oncology. "I didn't know the oncology unit wasn't required to adhere to the visiting hours. On 4 South, at 8:30 P.M. the visiting hours were over, and we asked everyone to leave. If they didn't, then security was called to remove them. I feel so bad . . . I wish I would have known . . ."

When she told Bob Fortin to leave, she pushed him over the edge. The stress from watching his wife suffer had been immense, and he had no intention of leaving her. He had the rest of his life to be without her . . . tonight, and the rest of the nights he had left, he would be with her.

"Ma'am, I'm staying right here with my wife . . ." he clearly stated.

"Sir, if you don't leave, I will have to call security . . ."

"You don't have enough damn security in this building to pry me away from my wife. Now would you get the hell out of here so we can sleep . . ."

Esther left the room, but returned shortly with two security officers. "Sir, you will have to leave now," the younger officer stated.

"I'm not going anywhere" Bob clearly stated.

"Sir, if you don't leave, we will call the police, and have you removed," the older security officer stated.

Becoming upset with their insensitivity to his plight, Bob quickly suggested, "why don't you use 9-1-1 to call the police, because anyone who tries to get me to leave will need emergency help . . ."

A few minutes later, a uniformed police officer entered the room, joined by the two security officers. "Sir," the police officer stated, "security has asked you to leave. If you don't, you will be arrested for criminal trespass."

"Officer, I have no intention of leaving my wife. If you don't get out so she can get some rest, I will throw you out . . . along with those pretend cops hiding behind you . . ."

With that, the police officer approached and grabbed Bob's arm. With an impressive military background, Bob Fortin was not about to be manhandled that easily. He quickly broke free from the police officers grip, pushing the officer back. When the young security officer lunged forward at him, Bob instinctively threw a strong left-hand punch that landed squarely on the security officer's nose, breaking it badly.

After a struggle that lasted less than a minute, but seemed like an hour, the police and security officers were able to get control of Bob. He was arrested, placed in handcuffs, and charged with multiple counts of battery, resisting arrest, disorderly conduct, and criminal trespass.

• • • • • • • • • •

The above incident is fictitious . . . or is it?

How many Esther Montore/Bob Fortin incidents occur regularly? Nobody can fault Bob for not wanting to leave the wife he loved so much. Can you fault the nurse, Esther Montore? Some will say yes; she should have known the rules. Others will say no, since it was obvious that nobody took time to explain the rules to her. Still others will fault her not because she didn't know how visiting hours were handled in the oncology unit but because of her hard-hearted approach with Bob Fortin.

Had she handled it differently . . . and she should have . . . the unfortunate outcome could have been avoided. Through her approach, Bob Fortin became defensive. He was forced beyond being verbally defensive, instead becoming physically violent with them. Yet the entire time, he felt he was in the defensive mode, feeling like he was the victim.

Too often, healthcare professionals see the technology and medicines at work but lose touch with the human side. The patients come and go, the diseases are the same, the doctors rant and rave, and somewhere in the middle of all this are the patients and their families.

When all is going well, everyone gets along fine. But when ideas, thoughts, or opinions differ, the end result is dictated by how the differences are handled.

The Aggression Continuum

One of the most critical steps in protecting yourself from the risk of physical violence is the ability to recognize the behavior patterns that lead to violence. Regardless of the amount of training you have, you are best prepared to protect yourself only when you are able to recognize progressive behavioral changes and to de-escalate the behavior back to a calm state. One of the most useful tools in recognizing these escalating behavior patterns is referred to as the *aggression continuum*. The aggression continuum represents the six stages that a person goes through on their way to violence.

To better appreciate the steps in the aggression continuum and to appreciate how one leads to another, imagine a six-step ladder (see Figure 4-1). The bottom step, where it is safest to stand, represents a state of calm. It is at this point that everyone is safe, and nobody's safety or well-being is jeopardized. Now visualize yourself climbing each step of the ladder with no one there to steady it. Each step gets progressively more dangerous. Suddenly, you have a decision to make. You're at that critical step where you have to decide whether to climb on to that top step, clearly labeled, "Caution: Do Not Stand on This Step." Remember, there is no one there to help steady the ladder, provide care if you fall, or even notify someone that you need help. This dangerous step on the ladder represents physical violence. Much like the person standing on the top step of that ladder, with no support or assistance, this is where the greatest risk of injury occurs. To be successful at de-escalating aggressive behavior, you must understand the aggression continuum and be able to identify behaviors associated with each step of this continuum, be able to understand the appropriate responses to de-escalate aggressive behaviors, and be able to restore a state of calm.

The six steps of the aggression continuum are the following:

1. Calm and nonthreatening
2. Verbally agitated
3. Verbally hostile
4. Verbally threatening
5. Physically threatening
6. Physically violent

At this point, it is important to look at each of the six steps individually and to recognize the behaviors that indicate the level of behavior on the continuum.

Figure 4-1 *Each step on the ladder represents a step on the aggression continuum. You never want your patient on the top step.*

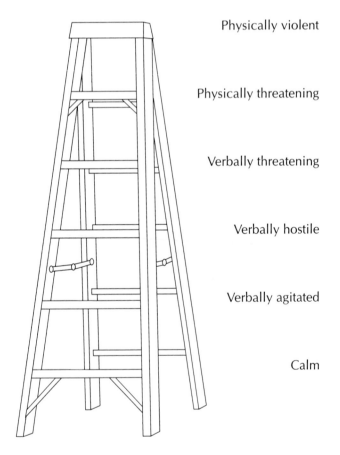

Physically violent

Physically threatening

Verbally threatening

Verbally hostile

Verbally agitated

Calm

Step 1: Calm and Nonthreatening

Calm is a state in which behaviors are easy for you to recognize and appreciate. Most of society spends its time in a state of calm, and most of the patients you treat will be calm and appreciative of your assistance. Calm patients will think logically and will understand the consequences of their actions.

When a person is calm their presence is nonthreatening. They do not present in any type of agitated manner. They interact with other people on a friendly, casual, or social basis. They are simply another person existing in society. It can not be overemphasized that this is the state that we always strive to restore. Our efforts should only cease when this state is resolved. Regardless of where a person is at on the aggression continuum, our goal is always the same—to restore a state of calm in the safest, most peaceful manner possible. It is also important to realize that a state of calm will always be restored. How it is restored from any given point on the continuum is the critical component.

Step 2: Verbally Agitated

The second step in our six-step continuum is a state in which the patient is verbally agitated. In this state, patients begin to express their anger with the situation or circumstances. This expression of anger is limited to verbal expressions only and is not directed at any person or object.

Compassionate human beings understand and appreciate the concept of verbal anger, because we have all experienced it. Think of an experience that recently upset you. Perhaps you were unable to find a tool you needed to complete a project at home. Maybe an outfit you planned on wearing to a social event wasn't clean. Maybe you went to the grocery store needing a particular item to prepare a meal, only to find they were out of the item. Any one of these situations may have caused you to mumble to yourself a few select words. You were not directing your anger at any person or object, rather you were merely expressing your displeasure with the situation in which you found yourself.

Imagine a cabinet containing several bottles of champagne. Individually, each bottle represents the state of calm. If one bottle of champagne is picked up and shaken, the pressure inside starts to build. When the cork is removed, the pressure is relieved, and the cork can soon be replaced and the bottle put back in storage. Imagine though what would happen if the cork weren't removed. The pressure inside the bottle would continue to expand until ultimately the bottle exploded. When it reached that point, it would likely damage the other bottles in the cabinet as well.

People are much the same as that bottle of champagne. For the most part, a person functions in a state of calm. Occasionally, like our bottle of champagne, a person is shaken up and the pressure inside builds. If the pressure is not relieved, like in the champagne bottle, the person will explode. But in the verbally agitated state, as people vent the built-up pressure, they normally return themselves to a state of calm with little or no intercession on your part. It is for this reason you must recognize the verbally agitated state and understand how to interact with patients to help bring them back to a state of calm. You don't want them to progress to the next step.

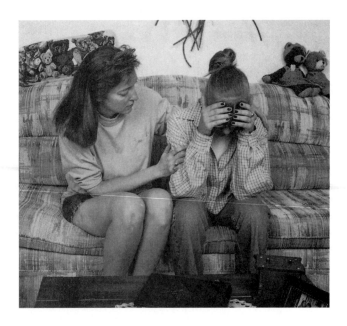

Figure 4-2 *Although the prehospital provider may be present, a family member may often be more helpful in calming an agitated loved one. In such cases, the prehospital provider should be an available resource at the scene and not the primary resource.*

Case Scenario
You are called to the residence of a 16-year-old female who has been threatening suicide since breaking up with a boyfriend. You are dispatched for a "female subject out of control." Upon arrival, your patient is sitting on the couch with her mother, crying. Her eyes are red and swollen, but she seems to be in control of herself now. After identifying yourself, the patient tells you she was devastated when she learned her boyfriend had broken up with her and "flipped out." Her mother tells you that she called 9-1-1 from her car after her daughter called her screaming and crying, saying she was going to kill herself. Your patient does not seem to be in any distress and wishes no assistance from you. She is calm and does not seem to be in any distress. After establishing that her parents will be staying with her, you contact your base hospital, and a medical refusal is granted.

Can you appreciate how this patient was verbally agitated. Upon learning that her boyfriend was breaking up with her, she reacted by "venting the pressure" while talking to her mother on the phone. Once the anger was vented, she returned to a state of calm, and with the assistance of her parents was able to cope with the situation. Can this patient carry out a threat of self-injury? Absolutely. At the same time, she is being left with an obviously caring family, the hospital has authorized her release, and at no time was she a threat to the safety of the prehospital providers.

Step 3: Verbally Hostile

The verbally hostile patient presents similarly to the verbally agitated patient; however, during the verbally hostile phase, patients are oblivious to all efforts to calm them.

Let's use our champagne bottle as an example again: when the cork was released the pressure inside the bottle vented until all of the pressure was relieved, and the bottle could safely be replaced. When a person makes the transition from verbally agitated to verbally hostile, the pressure does not seem to stop. They are still expressing their anger with the situation or circumstance they are dealing with, but in this step the venting fails to bring them back to a state of calm.

Although their anger is still not directed at any person or object, you must realize that when an abnormally long period of time has passed and the patient is still in an angry state, the patient is sending a strong message that they are escalating up the stepladder. You may not be in direct risk of harm but realize that the patient is one step closer to that top step on the ladder.

Case Scenario

Your engine company is called to assist an ambulance at a local shopping mall. On arrival, the ambulance crew is in the hallway outside a restaurant talking to a 26-year-old female. The dispatcher advises that you were called for assistance. The police were not immediately available, and the prehospital providers on the scene were concerned the individual might "go off." They have been on the scene for 20 minutes. The individual continues to voice anger "about nothing" and then quiets down, only to repeat the cycle. You learn she is on Ativan for an anxiety disorder but has not taken her medication for the past week. The individual is yelling about the government spying on her. She has not made any threats or shown any signs of aggression against any of those present. When the individual sees the dominating number of emergency service personnel on the scene, she willingly walks to the ambulance. She lies down on the cot and allows safety belts to be applied. She is transferred to the local hospital without incident.

Here, calming the patient down took considerable time. In Chapter 6, we will look at different techniques for de-escalating potentially violent behavior. The key factor in this example is that it took much longer for the patient to be calmed down and required a much greater effort than you anticipated.

Step 4: Verbally Threatening

In the next step the patient begins to direct his anger at a specific person or object. This may or may not include the prehospital provider who is there to help the person.

There are actually two very distinct clues that wave a red flag indicating the patient is reaching the fourth step on the stepladder. The first critical clue is that the patient will begin directing demands for action at you or others. For example, the patient may direct this statement toward you, "I want you to get the hell out of my house now." Or, they may direct the demand for action to someone else, such as "I want him to pay me the $50.00 he owes me and this will all be over with." The demand for specific action indicates that the patient has specific needs that he or she expects to have fulfilled. Demands for action by the patient is one of the simplest ways to recognize a verbally threatening person.

The second reliable clue is that the patient may indicate that there will be consequences if their demands are not met. This may include statements made to you such as: "I want you to get the hell out of my house now or I will throw you out myself." Or: "If he just pays me the $50.00 he owes me this will all be over. If he doesn't I am going to beat it out of him."

Again, an important point is that the patient is still in a verbal state. There are no direct physically aggressive moves made against you or anyone else present. At this point you must realize that you are at a critical point on the stepladder. *This is the last step in the verbal stages.* If not defused, the patient will continue into the physical stages. You *must* recognize verbally threatening statements, and the two common clues given in this state. If you fail to recognize these clues when a person becomes verbally threatening, or fail to take them seriously, there is a great likelihood that you could soon find yourself becoming the victim.

Case Scenario

You are called to a local tavern for an intoxicated male. Police are also en route. Upon arrival, you and the police approach a middle-aged man sitting alone at the bar. You are advised that he fell from a barstool and that the bartender was worried he had injured himself. As you gather information, you hear a commotion and observe the individual pointing his fingers at the police officer. The officer is trying to talk the individual down, but he continues to yell at him, "there ain't none of you big enough to get me to leave here . . . and I'll whip the ass of any of ya that try." The officer exercises professional restraint and continues to talk the individual down. The individual continues to tell the officer to "get the hell out of here before I stop being a nice guy." You hear numerous threats being made against the officer, and following his instructions, you leave the building and stage outside, as additional officers arrive. A few minutes later, police escort the individual, now in handcuffs, out of the building.

In this case, the prehospital providers were lucky. Police were on the scene and were willing to take responsibility and control of the individual. Remember, your role as a prehospital provider is not to engage in physical

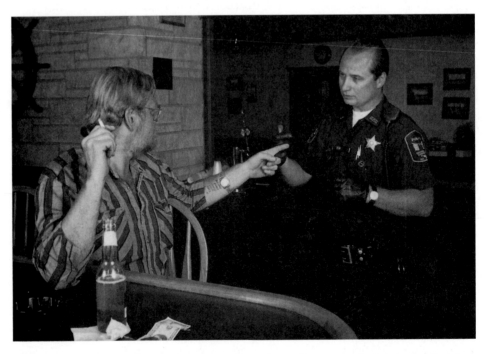

Figure 4-3 *Prehospital providers must allow the police to do their job, for their own safety as well as the safety of the patient and the police officer. Staging in a safe area until police have the situation secured is always advised.*

encounters but to provide care to the sick and injured. When an individual becomes verbally threatening, you must assess the situation and choose the best action. In this case, the best choice was to withdraw and allow the individuals with the best training and experience to perform their duties. But what if the police had not been present? How would you have handled the case? We will look at options in Chapter 6 when we discuss de-escalation techniques.

Step 5: Physically Threatening

When a patient reaches the fifth step in the continuum, you must realize that you have, for all intents and purposes, lost control of the situation. Physically threatening patients must be taken seriously, because they are now only one step away from the top step on our stepladder.

When patients become physically threatening, they will very likely quit voicing demands for action and threats of consequences. Instead, body language becomes a critical factor. Patients that are physically threatening will commonly take a physical stance that suggests violence. This may include making a fist, changing the position of their feet to better balance themselves, or making gestures suggestive of physical attack such as pounding a fist into a hand, or pumping a fist in the face of the prehospital provider. Any of these must be recognized as a prelude to violence.

You must also be aware that the patient who is at the fifth step may begin looking around the room for objects that can be used as weapons to strike out at you or anyone else present. We strongly advocate that when you are dealing with a patient in this state, you maintain close eye contact with the patient without entering into a staring contest. The eyes become the pathways to the mind. To the patient who is becoming physically threatening, more often than not, their eyes will tell you what their next move will be. Watch to see if they are scanning the area for a weapon. Are they sizing you up to determine how to overpower you? Are they looking at you for any possible weapons you may be carrying to use against them? It is again critical to recognize that while the eyes will usually telegraph the patient's actions, a stare down will likely push them over the edge.

Staring is a form of psychological cornering (we will talk more about cornering in Chapter 6). When a person feels cornered, there is usually only one way out and that is to fight. You must use every degree of caution and reason to avoid a stare down with the patient.

The physically threatening patient may also be trying to anticipate how prepared you are to deal with them if they become physically violent. They may make false gestures at you in an attempt to determine your response. Are you prepared to respond in a defensive mode? Does your body language indicate to the patient that you are an easy victim for him to take? Does your voice suggest fear or anxiety over dealing with the patient? Do you present an image of confidence to the patient? As much as you are sizing up the patient, the patient is also sizing you up. The key difference, however, is that you are sizing the patient up in order to de-escalate the situation and to perhaps switch to a form of physical self-defense or self-preservation. The patient is sizing you up for one simple reason: to overtake you. Are you prepared for the challenge?

Step 6: Physically Violent

Unfortunately, it has happened. Your attempts to de-escalate the situation have failed, and your patient now becomes physically violent. At this point all attempts to de-escalate cease, and your mode switches to one of self-defense and self-protection. Your goal now is to avoid being injured at the hands of your patient and to gain physical control without causing further harm or injury to him or her. This is a very fine line to walk and will require the use of physical force on your part.

Starting in Chapter 7, we will spend time discussing techniques of physical self-defense and physical takedowns. It is important to understand that laws on the amount of force that you may legally use will vary from state to state. Long before you find yourself in a position in which you are dealing with a physically violent patient, you must know to what degree you may use force. Most states are similar in that the degree of force allowed is usually the degree of force necessary to protect yourself from injury or death. Even though this may be the case in many states, this is not a legal opinion. It is recommended that you consult with legal council to obtain specific information on the laws on the use of force in your jurisdiction. Nothing could be worse than using force to protect yourself from injury and then to later find out that you exceeded your legal level of authority and could face criminal and/or civil charges.

Summary

Every healthcare provider must be able to defend him- or herself when the need arises. This is critical to personal safety and survival. Still, having to defend one's self against personal attack should be a last resort. Always maintain de-escalation of aggressive behavior and the restoration of calm before physical violence erupts as your primary goal.

The steps in the aggression continuum just introduced must be rehearsed over and over. To be effective, proficiency must be developed. The healthcare provider must be able to recognize behavior at each level in the continuum and to react accordingly. As was previously emphasized, the healthcare provider won't always have the luxury of starting at a state of calm and seeing the behavior escalate from that point. He or she may walk into a situation in which the behavior is already at the second or third level and must be able to react appropriately from that point.

Team Interventions

"I Had Been Taking Care of Him For So Long . . ."

"Get away from me . . . I'll kill you . . ."

Thurman L. Jackson was an impressive old man. At 81 years of age, he was a proud veteran of World War II and had served as an elite member of one of the Army's proudest team of soldiers. Even the 11 months he had spent in a prisoner of war camp hadn't broken his will or his spirit.

After the war, "Thurm" went on to become a masonry worker, eventually building a very successful construction business. He and his wife raised two children, a son and a daughter. Thurm and "Babe" were inseparable. In business and in life, they were the perfect partners, until her sudden death nine years earlier. Despite the heartbreaking loss of his life partner, Thurm seemed to be bouncing back. Then, within a year, he was forced to deal with yet another tragedy. His son, Jerry, a successful accountant and father of four, was killed by a drunk driver while driving home late one evening.

Jerry's death was more than Thurm could cope with. Some said it was the real reason that, within another few months, he suffered a major stroke. After the stroke, his daughter tried bringing him home to live with her own family. But the stroke left him partially paralyzed, and more so, the change in his mental cognition was obvious. He saw imaginary people and often seemed so confused that he thought his daughter and her family were old friends from his young days.

Placing him in a nursing home was no easy decision, but everyone knew it was the right one. Thurm needed more care than he could receive in his daughter's home, and she had concerns about him being alone around the children. The Garden View Care Center seemed perfect . . . clean, bright, cheerful . . . nothing like one might expect a nursing home to be.

The staff of the nursing home enjoyed having Thurm there. Most of the time, he was cheerful and it was a pleasure to care for him. On occasions, such as now, he seemed to be in another world. But he had never become violent.

When Jenna Wilson, a nurse's aide with three years experience walked into his room, she knew something was wrong. Thurm was standing with his back against the wall, holding his cane as if it were a sword. "Thurm, what's wrong . . . ?"

"How did you know my name . . . I didn't tell you my damn name . . ."

Jenna knew Thurm had been a POW in the war, but she had known him for a long time and always took care of him. Surely he would recognize her.

"I'm warning you . . . I'll kill all of you . . ."

As Jenna approached him, he seemed to get more apprehensive, drawing his cane up in front of him, holding it like a weapon.

Momentarily, Jenna thought about calling for help. She knew how strong people . . . even the elderly . . . could become when they were upset. But Thurm was *her pal . . . she sure didn't want to risk him getting hurt. She would just talk to him until he settled down.*

"Thurm, it's me, Jenna . . . your nurse."

"I'm warning you . . . stay back damn you . . ."

"Thurm, lets go outside," she spoke softly, approaching him and extending her hand.

Then it happened. Without further warning, Thurm swung the cane, striking Jenna in the head. Stunned, Jenna froze. Again and again, he struck her with the cane. Jenna felt the blood rushing down her face. Soon the pain from the repeated blows seemed to fade. The room suddenly seemed loud and started spinning.

"Stay awake . . . don't fall out . . ." she told herself. It was no use. The blows continued until she lost consciousness.

Later, in a hospital bed, Jenna learned that a maintenance worker walked by and saw Thurm beating the floor with his cane. The maintenance worker was unable to see Jenna from the door, since she was on the floor next to the bed. When he walked into the room, he saw Jenna lying in a pool of blood. With the assistance of several others, the cane was taken from Thurm, and he was taken from the room.

● ● ● ● ● ● ● ● ● ●

Jenna was off work for 11 weeks. She suffered a severe concussion and head lacerations that took 137 stitches to close. Even after the physical wounds healed, Jenna continued to suffer headaches and was unable to drive. Holding her young daughter was a chore. This was not what she wanted from caring for the elderly.

No matter how well a healthcare provider knows or thinks he or she knows the residents or patients, personal safety cannot be forsaken. There is no guarantee that Thurm could have been disarmed without injury to anyone. But certainly, if there truly were "safety in numbers" then a team approach would have lessened the chances of injury.

Prevention and Response Strategies

Responding to violence is dangerous enough. Add to it the issues of violence faced by healthcare providers discussed in Chapter 2 plus the need to look out for the welfare of the "victim/perpetrator" of violence, and the waters really get muddied. Some say healthcare providers should never be allowed to strike an individual, regardless of the circumstances. Others say healthcare providers shouldn't even be allowed to temporarily restrain a patient—not even for the safety of the patient, the provider, or others. Due to the litigious society in which we live, few people will go on record as saying that healthcare providers have a right to protect themselves from a violent patient. The content in this text is based on prevention and response strategies, teaching the reality that no matter how much you plan and implement prevention methods, violence can and does occur frequently in your chosen profession. To minimize the likelihood of violence and to increase the odds of handling every situation effectively, the team approach is the safe and logical approach to take.

This philosophy is not unique and sounds much simpler than it is. It is based on the notion that every individual has the right of self-protection, including healthcare providers. The healthcare provider, like those in every other profession, has a job to do. Their job, however, involves dealing with every kind and type of person society has to offer, from the extremely affluent politician, singer, dancer, or movie star, to the lowest forms of life imaginable—child molesters, murderers, rapists, spouse abusers, and so on. Healthcare providers see and do things most people could never even imagine. Yet they are expected to remain professional and in control of their feelings and emotions at all times, to protect and treat the patient, regardless of who it is, and to put themselves in danger, often without the same guarantee of protection that average citizens are afforded. Not a simple task for even the most seasoned professional.

Many people will agree that a healthcare provider's primary mission should be to help with the healing process of patients. Many also subscribe to the belief that every individual has a basic right to defend themselves against violence. Still, industry standards seldom condone the use of physical intervention and restraint, except under extreme circumstances that include the following:

Patient Protection
Many patients, both prehospital and those hospitalized, have a tendency to become violent for the reasons discussed in earlier chapters. Some tend to lash out by trying to harm themselves, whether intentionally or involuntarily, whether conscious or unconscious. Healthcare providers, in our opinion, not only have a right to protect the patient from him- or herself, but a responsibility as well, which may involve the use of physical intervention and/or restraint. However, the amount of physical intervention should be the least amount necessary to protect the patient, but, at the same time, needs to be enough to keep others from being hurt in the process.

Provider Protection
As discussed earlier, healthcare providers have a job to do and this involves a wide range of different types of people. The healthcare provider should do this job in the most caring and compassionate manner possible. He or she should be highly skilled and meticulously trained to perform necessary duties, without needlessly putting themselves in harm's way. The fact that an individual sustained a head injury, has emotional problems, or became infected with a disease is, of course, tragic. Nevertheless, these conditions should not prohibit the healthcare provider from the basic right to self-protection. While they must be compassionate in their response to all these individuals, they also owe it to their family, friends, other patients, and co-workers to maintain some semblance of safety for themselves.

Innocent Bystander Protection
Once a patient is under the care of a healthcare provider, the healthcare provider becomes responsible for ensuring the safety of the patient and any bystanders. This is not to say the healthcare provider assumes responsibility for the actions of the patient, only that she or he should take reasonable steps to ensure that the patient causes no harm. This may or may not involve the use of physical intervention and/or restraint. On a case-by-case basis, the circumstances will dictate the actions of the healthcare provider.

Property Protection
This tends to get a little more criticism from those who believe every situation can be handled without physical intervention or restraint. One common argument is "property can be replaced, people can't." While this is true, think about the damage a single patient could cause without any inter-

vention to protect property. In the back of an ambulance, a patient left alone could destroy property, cause an accident, destroy lifesaving/life-sustaining equipment, or cause irreparable damage to the ambulance itself, thereby taking it out of service for a matter of hours or even days. Likewise, in a hospital, the patient left to destroy property could do many of the same things listed above, as well as take the caregiver's time and attention away from critical patients who need the care the most.

Again, these may sound simple; however, each situation is unique and presents new challenges for the healthcare provider. For example, what happens when the disruptive patient is a 10 year old or an 85 year old? What happens when the patient is a healthy 20 year old and the health-care provider is near retirement? What about the patient who is armed or is in close proximity to a number of items that could be used as weapons? What if there are several family members near the patient and only one healthcare provider? Or, what if there are five or six healthcare providers and only one patient?

Each situation must be looked at individually before any physical intervention techniques or restraints are used. That is one reason risk management professionals discourage policies that severely limit the actions of the healthcare provider. Policies need to be written in a way that allow healthcare providers to choose from options, depending on the circumstances, rather than dictate a prescribed course of action. For the remainder of this chapter, and throughout your career, keep the following basic tenets on the use of physical intervention and/or restraint in mind:

1. Never use any type of physical intervention or restraint unless it is legal and absolutely necessary to protect the patient, the caregiver, bystanders, or property.
2. Use only the least amount of physical intervention and/or restraint necessary based on the total circumstances of the situation.
3. Use only the amount of intervention and/or restraint that any other reasonable person in the same situation would use.
4. Know and follow local, state, and national laws on the use of physical intervention and restraints in your jurisdiction as well as your own company policy.
5. Anticipate and prepare *as a team* to confront violence. Odds are significant that if you are in the healthcare field long enough, you will be face-to-face with a violent patient at some point in your career.

The Role of the Team

The role of the violence response/prevention team can be as little or as much as you desire. The violence response/prevention team should carefully consider each of the following responsibilities:

1. To assess:
   a. Current policies, procedures, standards, and practices for vulnerabilities to incidents of violence
   b. Past records of injury/incidents for patterns of violence:
      1) Does violence occur more during certain times of the day?
      2) Does violence occur more during certain days of the week?
      3) Does violence occur more during holidays?
      4) Does violence occur more in certain areas of the city? Of the facility?

5) Does violence occur more when staffing is at its lowest? Or perhaps at its highest?
6) Does violence occur more when certain staff are working?
7) Is there a history of patients who have been violent in the past?
8) Are there any recognizable trends that could be managed by changes in staffing, changes in procedures, implementation of protective devices, etc.

c. The physical plant
1) Are there areas of the building, ambulance, or city that are unsafe due to inadequate lighting?
2) Distance from help?
3) Lack of protective devices?
4) Other unsafe or hazardous conditions?

d. Training needs
1) Is staff adequately trained to the level needed based on the type of incidents occurring in your jurisdiction?
2) Has staff received training in verbal de-escalation?
3) Has staff received training in physical self-defense, including the use of seclusion and restraints?

2. To define:
a. Policies, procedures, and practices that need to be added or changed to competently handle aggression
b. Protective equipment needed in the event of an emergency
c. The role of the healthcare provider when confronted by violence
d. The responsibilities of the healthcare provider when confronted by violence
e. Options and assistance available to the healthcare provider when confronted by violence
f. The role of the dispatcher to minimize the likelihood of violence and/or increase awareness for the healthcare provider
g. The training needs of the healthcare provider and all ancillary personnel who might be confronted by violence

3. To implement:
a. Policies, procedures, and practices that have been added or changed
b. The use of protective equipment
c. Training in aggression management and response to include:
1) Verbal de-escalation skills
2) One-on-one confrontations
3) Team intervention procedures
d. Regular security inspections
e. Regular meetings at predefined intervals to review the following:
1) The effect of policies and procedures on violence prevention and injury reduction
2) Results of security inspections
3) Incidents of violence with or without injury
a) What could have prevented the incident?
b) Was it handled properly?
c) What, if anything, will be done differently in the future?
4) Patterns of violence
5) Future prevention strategies

Many hospitals, fire departments, and ALS/BLS services make these meetings a part of their existing environment of care/safety committee activity.

4. To recommend/assist with:
   a. Community violence prevention programs
   b. School violence prevention programs
   c. Public/private law enforcement liaison meetings

The Team vs. the Individual

Why all of the emphasis on team intervention procedures? The reasons are numerous, and include those listed below:

1. The visibility and presence of more than one person often serve as a deterrent to an individual contemplating an aggressive action.
2. Based on their experience and training, team members provide an extra set of eyes and ears to watch and listen for unknown hazards.
3. There are increased avenues for communication. While one person is communicating with the patient, another may communicate with the police, the dispatcher, another staff member, another family member, and so on.
4. Properly trained teams are less likely to use force, thereby reducing the likelihood of injury to the provider as well as the patient.
5. Team members may have individual attributes that contribute to the whole of the team, such as, one person may excel at verbal intervention while another excels in physical techniques. Not only will working together increase the confidence of each individual, but it also increases the odds of safely intervening without the use of force, which should always be the goal.
6. Working together as a team provides witnesses that are able to defend the actions taken based on the total circumstances of the situation rather than the emotional testimony of the patient's friends and relatives. (Keep in mind that if you are not acting in the best interest of the patient and the team, team members may also be called upon to present testimony against you.)
7. After an incident, team members can share ideas and strategies on ways to prevent future occurrences.

Preparing the Team

The first step in preparing the team is to decide on the level of their involvement. Go through the previous list and identify in whole, or in part, the responsibilities of the team. Once the team responsibilities are determined, management must commit the resources needed to make the team effective. Resources include, but are not limited to the following:

- Cost of equipment and supplies
- Cost of training the team to a competent level
- Salaries of team members for meetings, training classes, research projects, and other like expenses

The next step is to solicit the cooperation and involvement of team members. This should be a voluntary team. People who are mandated to serve on a team may resent being there and may not put forth the effort required to make it effective. Many organizations offer incentives to encourage involvement. Again, any offer of incentives should be done after voluntary assignments are given. This is not to suggest that the only people who are trained in violence prevention are the team members. All staff should be trained to handle violent incidents safely and effectively. The team should be trained in these areas as well as in the extra duties listed previously.

Finally, with the requirements in place and the team selected, establish a training program for the members of the team. This may be done by local law enforcement, security experts, in-house staff, or aggression management experts. Whichever you choose, carefully check the credentials of the "expert." Use qualified aggression management experts to get you started. They should be well versed in laws on the use of force, the use of restraint and seclusion, and verbal de-escalation. Often, they will leave you with an assessment tool for conducting your own inspections throughout the year.

Team training should include, at a minimum:

1. Security assessment procedures
2. Quality improvement procedures
3. Pre-planning the safest way to deal with a potentially violent person
4. Advance recognition of impending violence
5. Verbal de-escalation techniques
6. Realistic, proven physical intervention methods that include:
   a. One-on-one confrontations
   b. Team intervention
   c. Physical intervention techniques that allow you to gain control of the situation using the least amount of force possible
   d. Liability issues surrounding the use of force and physical restraint
7. Basic defensive tactics, including:
   a. Proper body mechanics
   b. Proper approach toward the violent subject
   c. Proper distancing techniques
   d. Verbal direction
   e. Blocking and impact techniques
   f. Takedowns
8. Restraint techniques, including:
   a. Review of the types and styles available
   b. Selection of the right type for the situation
   c. Best method of application
   d. Laws governing their proper use and application
   e. Departmental policy governing their proper use and application
9. Edged weapons defense
10. Armed violence defense

The Team's Response

Now that the team is assembled and has been properly trained, how do they respond? Remember that there is safety in numbers. Intervening alone is dangerous. A team of two or more people will provide a safer approach for everyone, including the patient.

Obtain Assistance as Soon as Violence Is Anticipated

Team members, police, security, or other assistance should be summoned quickly and discreetly. Nonessential personnel and bystanders will only add to the confusion. Team members (as needed) may be staged in an area proximal to the location of the incident.

Attempt De-escalation Techniques

- Maintain adequate distance.
- Move toward a safe location, if possible.
- Explain that you are there to help.
- Monitor your composure, remain in control, and be confident.
- Maintain a nonthreatening posture.
- Distract the attention of the aggressor by conversing in a calm tone.
- Acknowledge the patient's concerns and feelings.
- If applicable, ask for weapon(s) to be placed on the ground (not handed over).

Determine Who Is in Charge of the Team

This is an area in which many teams get into trouble. Too often, someone's ego gets in the way of rational thinking. The team leader is often the first person on the scene, or a person who has established rapport with the patient. Still, as a general rule of thumb, the person in charge is the one who is "closest" to the danger zone.

For example, you arrive at the scene of a domestic dispute. Upon arrival, the battered wife is standing toe-to-toe with her husband. You are expected to take control of the situation and to provide care to the wife. You begin to approach and get about five feet away when the husband tells you to stop or someone will get hurt. Who is in charge at this point? The answer, in its simplest form, is the wife. She is the one within the danger zone of the threat. Many times, a third party, in an effort to assist, will try to take control of the situation, unknowingly causing an escalation of the incident and injury to the person in the danger zone. None of us, as healthcare providers, wants to be responsible for causing an incident to escalate. You've already summoned assistance, and as long as the husband and wife are not getting physically violent, wait for the assistance.

The following real-life dramatization depicts what is meant by third-party interference:

> Security was summoned to the emergency department at the local hospital. Upon arrival, security observed a male patient, still in a hospital gown, walking backward toward the sliding glass exit doors. He was followed by two nurses, walking slowly and attempting to reason with the patient about why he had to stay and receive treatment. Security joined the two nurses and convinced the patient to return to his room. Since they all were standing in front of the sliding glass doors with motion sensors, the doors kept opening and closing. As security and the two nurses approached the patient to assist him back to his room, another hospital worker approached and reached over the patient's head to turn off the doors. The worker's intention was to keep the doors from opening and closing. The patient apparently took it as an aggressive move toward him and began to fight. The patient then had to be subdued and physically restrained to keep from hurting himself, the staff, and the bystanders in the nearby waiting room.

With proper team training, the whole confrontation could have been avoided. The worker who attempted to shut off the doors would have known not to approach unless directed by another team member. This is just one example of how a third party can cause a situation to escalate needlessly. Can you think of one, or more, which have happened to you?

Like any team, violence response teams need to practice. Conduct regular drills. They are the best way to improve effectiveness. Use real-life situations as your drill. Train participants to be as realistic as possible in their reactions; however, the primary rule should be, nobody gets hurt. Don't surprise law enforcement or other healthcare organizations with your "unannounced" drill. Always get their cooperation ahead of time.

Use your experience during drills and during real-life situations as a basis for debriefing sessions. In the debriefing, focus on what went right, what went wrong, what could have been better, and how to improve next time. In addition, the debriefing should include all staff and patients, including bystanders, involved with the incident. Facilitate discussion about the following:

✓ What happened
✓ What factors contributed to or caused the incident
✓ Each person's role in the incident
✓ Any personal feelings or facts of concern

Summary

A team approach to aggression management affords benefits that individual responses cannot. These include various protections for the patient, the caregiver, and bystanders, including the patient's family and friends, as well as protection for property that is proximal to the incident, regardless of ownership.

Regardless of the size or strength of the team, physical intervention should always be viewed as a last resort. Every verbal de-escalation technique available should be tried before physical intervention is used. If physical intervention becomes necessary, then only the amount of force necessary to regain control of the situation should be used. Always remember the "reasonable person" standard.

The structure of violence response teams may vary among organizations, but the role is generally the same. Common roles of the team include risk assessments, development and implementation of policies and procedures, providing advise, counsel, and training to the organization, and of course, incident responses.

Defusing Aggressive Behavior

"What Would You Do?"

Take a look at each of the scenarios below, and choose the response that best describes how you would react.

After completing all five scenarios, score your answers using the guidelines at the end.

Scenario 1

You are called to the psych unit to assist in defusing a potentially violent situation. When you arrive on the unit, the patient is backed into a corner, his arms curled in front of him. The nursing staff tells you that he will become violent if anyone tries to come near him. What would you do?

   a. Call for assistance, approach him, and grab his arms so he can't hit you.
   b. Call for assistance and hope a show of force will intimidate the patient.
   c. Keep a safe distance, and calmly talk to the patient in a nonthreatening manner.
   d. Inform the patient what you expect from him, and tell him what the consequences will be if he does not comply.

Scenario 2

Your ambulance is dispatched to a known drug house for a possible overdose. En route to the scene, police tell you that they do not have an officer on the scene and aren't sure if the situation is secured. Do you:

   a. Proceed in and approach the house with your "guard up."
   b. Stop, turn around, and return to quarters until police advise you to proceed in.
   c. Park in front of the residence and wait for police.
   d. Stage a safe distance away, and wait for police to arrive at the scene and assure you that it is secured.

Scenario 3

You are a nurse on an Alzheimer's unit in a large nursing home. Dealing with combative residents is "routine." Over a period of time, you find yourself becoming less and less patient with the residents, especially when they are very confused and resist your efforts to help them. Your temper is growing shorter, and you worry that you may become abusive with them out of frustration. What would you feel is your best response?

   a. Continue to work, and work through the hostility.
   b. Meet with the director of nursing or administrator, and ask to be assigned elsewhere.
   c. Meet with the director of nursing or the administrator, and ask for access to the Employee Assistance Program and for reassignment to another unit.
   d. Resign and hope to find work in a similar field that doesn't involve an Alzheimer's unit.

Scenario 4

The emergency department is busy, and the last thing you need is another drunk, especially one in police custody. Two chest pains, a stroke patient, a child hit by a car, and three lacerations waiting to be sutured is more than enough in a small emergency department like this one. But the drunk doesn't seem to understand that his timing is less than impeccable and decides to impress you with his knowledge of profane words as you try to do an initial assessment. Since that doesn't impress you, he decides to try and get up to prove to you that he can "leave any stinkin' time he wants." Your best response is to:

   a. Stay with him and try to reason him down, even if he continues to become more assertive with you.

   b. Place him into leather restraints since he has threatened to leave and is in police custody.

   c. Call security and allow them to get him under control so a proper medical assessment can be performed.

   d. Call the police and have them come in and watch him, since he is their "guest."

Scenario 5

You are called to a local drinking establishment to treat a subject who has been struck in the head with a beer bottle. Upon arrival, police have a male, approximately 25 years old, pinned on the front terrace of the business. He is face down and is in handcuffs. You notice that his feet are also shackled, and ankle cuffs have been secured to his wrist cuffs. He continues to cuss at the police, and you notice the blood on his forehead. The police sergeant tells you to get your stretcher and take him in like this . . . that the cuffs aren't coming off. Your best action is to:

   a. Take the ranking officer aside and explain to him why the patient can't be transported in this position.

   b. Set your own restraints up in advance, then place the patient on the stretcher, and secure him in your restraints, one limb at a time, without police assistance.

   c. Transport him in the position in which the police have him.

   d. Have police transport him in a police car in that position.

Score your responses as follows:

Scenario 1		**Scenario 4**	
Choice a:	0 points	Choice a:	2 points
Choice b:	2 points	Choice b:	0 points
Choice c:	10 points	Choice c:	10 points
Choice d:	5 points	Choice d:	5 points
Scenario 2		**Scenario 5**	
Choice a:	5 points	Choice a:	10 points
Choice b:	0 points	Choice b:	2 points
Choice c:	2 points	Choice c:	0 points
Choice d:	10 points	Choice d:	0 points
Scenario 3			
Choice a:	0 points		
Choice b:	5 points		
Choice c:	10 points		
Choice d:	2 points		

So how did you do? If you scored 40 to 50 points, you did great. You should be able to recognize situations that place you at risk and be able to take the appropriate steps to protect yourself and to defuse the behavior.

If you scored less than 40, you are encouraged to read Chapter 6 very carefully and perhaps more than once. Recognizing potentially violent behavior is the first critical component, but being able to defuse the behavior is equally critical. Remember, the goal is to always restore a state of calm.

Introduction

In Chapter 4, we identified the six steps of our aggression continuum, listed below:

1. Calm and nonthreatening
2. Verbally agitated
3. Verbally hostile
4. Verbally threatening
5. Physically threatening
6. Physically violent

In this chapter, we will look at the steps on the continuum and also at that response by the healthcare provider that will help diffuse the aggressive behavior and return the patient to a state of calm.

Calm and Nonthreatening Behavior

When dealing with a patient who is calm and nonthreatening the provider seldom finds him- or herself at any risk of personal injury at the hands of the patient. Assuming that the provider provides proper medical treatment, this should remain true throughout the entire period that the prehospital provider has contact with the patient. When dealing with the patient who is calm and nonthreatening, the provider should focus on specific goals designed to meet the needs of the patient while maintaining a state of calm.

Provide Quality Medical Care

We previously established that the calm and nonthreatening patient is the type of patient with which the provider will most frequently have contact. When dealing with this type of patient, the provider is focused on the immediate medical and emotional needs of the patient and/or the family and friends who may be present at the scene. Providing quality medical care and stabilizing the patient is the goal of the prehospital provider. By focusing on the needs of the patient, following appropriate medical protocols, and communicating with the patient and family members as to what is being done to help the patient and why, the prehospital provider can often avoid any escalation of aggression by those who may be present at the scene, including the patient.

Respect the Patient's Dignity

Oftentimes, prehospital providers are called to a scene and find the patient in what may be described as a compromising position. Experienced providers can identify with some of these conditions. Many times patients are found, for example, in showers or bathtubs, on the bathroom floor, or in bed. Additionally, when the prehospital provider is called to a person's home, the house may be unkempt, messy, or even trashed. Prehospital providers often find a person in their worst moments. He or she must always remember that their role is to provide emergency medical care and not to pass judgment on how other people live. Regardless of the person's physical appearance at the time, or the condition in which they are found, the prehospital provider must always remember to respect the dignity of that individual as a human being, to provide for their medical needs, and to treat all patients the same regardless of status or class. Respect for human dignity must be the trademark of the provider, despite the situation. Patient modesty, regardless of gender, should always be addressed by covering the exposed patient with a sheet or blanket.

Listen to Patient Concerns

Providing routine medical care to the patient often becomes second nature to the provider. This is especially true in cases that are of a common and frequent nature, such as taking vital signs, splinting, and immobilizing. The professional healthcare provider is able to provide this type of treatment almost subconsciously. Having performed these skills over and over, it is easy for the provider to assume that the patient and everyone else at the scene are familiar with the procedures and skills being used. Although performing the skills may be second nature to the provider, for most patients it is a new experience. Providers must always remember to communicate to patients exactly what they are going to do whenever possible. Assuming that your patient is medically stable and time and surroundings permit, allow the patient the opportunity to ask questions. Be sure to tell the patient what you are going to do in advance. If the patient expresses concern over the treatment being provided and circumstances permit, explain to the patient why the treatment is necessary. If the provider approaches the patient and begins applying practical skills without informing the patient, he or she may very well act defensively. The patient will want to know what is being done to them and why before allowing the provider to proceed. Once the patient has become defensive, they may very well move onto the next step of the ladder. Listening to patient concerns and communicating effectively may be the provider's two best skills, even if he or she is very good at patient medical management.

Be Compassionate and Caring

Simple as this may sound, it is often more difficult than we want to admit. When caring for an elderly patient who may have fallen and sustained a hip fracture, most providers exercise compassion, skill, and a caring attitude. Unfortunately, that is not always the case when the prehospital provider is dealing with a patient who does not appreciate their efforts or may not necessarily want the prehospital provider to be present. A compassionate and caring approach when managing this type of patient is one of the most effective tools to diffuse any type of escalating behavior. Regardless of where the person is on the continuum, a caring and compassionate attitude will often prove to be a successful step in de-escalation.

Verbally Agitated Behavior

You will recall that when we talked about the verbally agitated patient in Chapter 4, we compared that person to a champagne bottle. When the champagne bottle is shaken, the pressure builds up inside. When the cork is removed, the pressure can vent to the point at which the cork can be replaced and the bottle put back into storage. When dealing with the verbally agitated patient, the provider should always keep the image of the champagne bottle in mind. Since the verbally agitated patient is not directing his or her anger at any specific person or object, there are some simple techniques that the provider can use to help bring that patient back to a state of calm.

Listen to the Patient

Too often, *we hear but we don't listen*. The verbally agitated patient is using verbal expression to vent the pressure that is built up inside of them. By taking time and listening to the patient, the provider allows the patient the opportunity to de-escalate him- or herself. Once the patient has vented their anger, the provider will begin to see the patient returning to a state of calm. All the provider has done is to listen and acknowledge the patient's feelings. The provider must be cautious not to interject personal biases or opinions when allowing the patient to vent their verbal anger. Many times the providers, with good intentions, begin to engage in conversation with a verbally agitated patient and will try to share opinions or personal experiences in an attempt to gain the trust and confidence of the patient. Unfortunately, the patient's opinion may differ from that of the provider's, and this may only lead to more agitation. Listening to the verbally agitated patient means giving them the time they need to place themselves back into a state of calm.

Respect the Patient

In most cases, your patient will be a good person. When the incident is over, your patient will want his or her self-respect and dignity intact. In addition, they not only will *want* their self-respect and dignity intact, they *deserve* to have them left intact. Your role as a healthcare professional is to help the patient work through the problem and allow the issue to resolve in such a way that no one is injured and that the patient feels good about him- or herself after the incident is over.

Remember that respect is a basic human need. Giving your patients the respect they deserve and not judging the things you hear or see will often help your efforts to restore or maintain a state of calm. At the very least, it will not add any more fuel to the fire.

Save the Patient's Self-Esteem

Healthcare providers reading this book will certainly have encountered a verbally agitated patient at some point in their career. The degree of agitation involved may vary, but once the patient has vented their anger and returned to a state of calm, he or she is again a reasonable person.

The provider must realize that once the episode is over, the patient deserves to be allowed to maintain their self-respect and self-esteem. The provider must also consider that the verbally agitated patient who is reacting to some type of stressor is probably not a bad person. Instead, he or she is a person who is having difficulty dealing with whatever the situation may be. Talking down to the patient, or making them feel bad or guilty about the behaviors they have displayed, or the comments they have made, will work against the caregiver's efforts to de-escalate the situation.

DO NOT Give Orders

Giving orders to the verbally agitated patient is almost a guaranteed step up on the ladder. Because the verbally agitated patient is not directing verbal anger at the provider, why would the provider want to order specific behaviors from a patient? The verbally agitated patient does not need to be spoken to in a condescending manner. They need to be listened to. None of us like to be given orders. Whether it is by a supervisor, a spouse, a partner, or anyone else, we are usually more willing to do things if we are asked to do them. If this is true during a state of calm, you can imagine how it impacts a verbally agitated person, especially when the one giving orders is a stranger who has now approached them with the intent of helping them. Someone once said: "People are like ropes. If you pull them, they will follow you anywhere. If you push them, they will go nowhere." How true a statement this is. The verbally agitated patient, already dealing with a difficult situation, will be much more likely to cooperate with the provider when they are given choices, as opposed to commands, on how to behave and act.

Verbally Hostile Behavior

The verbally hostile patient presents behavior similar to the verbally agitated patient. The big difference between these two steps on the ladder is that the verbally hostile patient is oblivious to all efforts to calm them. Again, how the provider deals with the patient will often dictate which direction the patient's behavior takes on the ladder.

When dealing with the verbally hostile patient, keep the following goals in mind.

Maintain a Nonthreatening Body Posture

The provider must be aware of his or her body language and the nonverbal signals that they are sending to the patient. This is especially true when looking at body posture. If the provider's posture is one that suggests physical contact or physical aggression, the patient may very well react in the same manner. Unfortunately, the provider in this case has used nonverbal signals to provoke the patient.

Instead, the provider should maintain a nonthreatening posture. Referred to as the *initial interview position,* this position allows the provider to verbally interact with the patient without sending any type of physical or threatening nonverbal signals.

In assuming the initial interviewing position, the provider stands with feet even and slightly more than shoulder width apart. The knees are slightly bent to help maintain balance. The hands are kept elevated, normally at chest height, allowing the patient to see that the provider holds no weapons or objects that could be used against the patient. Oftentimes, this is the position we normally take when dealing with other people. We assume this position without even realizing it. The position is nonthreatening, and conveys a signal that the prehospital provider is there to help the patient and not to harm them (see Figure 6-1).

Respect the Buffer Zone

Imagine that you are sitting in a classroom taking a refresher class. The instructor is going through a slide presentation, using a remote control to advance the slides. During the entire presentation, the instructor is standing directly behind your chair. After a period of time, you will likely start to feel uncomfortable, because the instructor is invading your space.

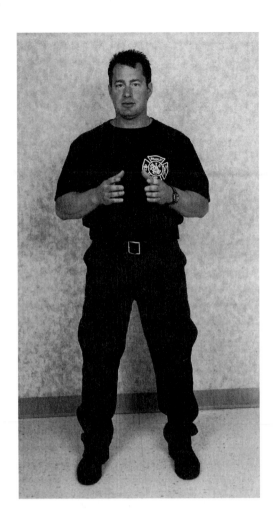

Figure 6-1 *The initial interview position allows the provider to interact with others without sending any threatening body signals.*

The verbally hostile patient experiences the same feelings. Without realizing it, the provider may position him- or herself in such a way that the patient begins to feel that his space is invaded. Unknowingly, the provider may be pushing the patient up the ladder.

There are many different schools of thought on the amount of space to maintain between the patient and the provider. Some defensive tactics instructors recommend an automatic buffer zone of 6 feet. Others advocate 8 feet, 10 feet, and some even 12 feet. Still others suggest that the buffer zone should be the equivalent of the patient's leg length plus an additional 1 or 2 feet. To determine the adequate buffer zone, the provider must take the conditions of the patient and the environment in which he or she is working into consideration. If the patient is sitting in a chair, the provider may be able to move closer to the patient while still maintaining a safe buffer zone. If the patient's body language is suggesting imminent physical aggression, then certainly the provider is going to be well-advised to maintain a greater buffer zone. There is no hard and fast rule on how large of a buffer zone to maintain. The provider must also take into consideration the medical needs of the patient. It is difficult enough to assess a patient who is verbally hostile. It is even more difficult to do so from 10 or 12 feet away. The provider must exercise common sense and good judgment when talking with the patient about an appropriate buffer zone. Observe the patient. Is the patient holding anything that could be used as a weapon against the prehospital provider? What about the physical environment? Is there anything near the patient that he or she could grab and use as a weapon? What about past knowledge of this patient? Have the providers had previous encounters with this patient? If so, was physical force necessary? Did the patient exhibit signs of physical aggression? These are all indicators that the provider must take into consideration when establishing the buffer zone. Proper positioning can be one of the provider's most effective self-defense tools. Always position yourself near an exit, in case a quick egress becomes necessary. And never allow yourself to be placed into a corner, where a safe escape may be impossible.

Keep Instructions Minimal

Instead of giving the patient directives or orders, give them choices. Allow the patient to understand that actions taken are directly related to the choices he or she makes. Again, as when dealing with the verbally agitated patient, the provider will find the verbally hostile patient much more receptive to requests than to orders.

Verbally Threatening Behavior

Previously, we established that the verbally threatening patient directs his or her anger toward another specific person; this may or may not include the provider. The provider must be able to recognize two very distinct clues that indicate that the patient is stepping toward the fourth step (verbally threatening) on the ladder. The first clue is that the patient begins to direct demands for action at the hospital provider or others at the scene. The second clue is that the patient may state that there will be consequences to deal with if their demands are not met. The provider must be aware that the situation is changing for the worse and that the patient is at the last step in the verbal portion of the aggression continuum. If the provider is not able to de-escalate this situation, the next step will become physical.

While it is more difficult to de-escalate the verbally threatening patient, the following are certain techniques that the provider can use successfully.

Maintain Eye Contact

This is not a situation in which the provider wants to turn his or her back on the patient or allow any attention to be diverted away from the patient. It has been said that the eyes are "the pathway to the soul." Normally, a person's eyes will dictate their next move. If the provider is able to maintain eye contact with the patient, very likely they may be able to anticipate the patient's next move and prepare for it in advance. Do not engage, however, in a staring contest with the patient. Some behaviorists suggest that attention be focused to the person's left eye, because it is the left side of the brain that receives and processes information. The provider may also find success by asking questions that end with the letters "<u>n't</u>." For example, if the provider wants to check the patient's vital signs, which of the following two approaches do you think would be more successful?

a) *Mr. Jones, why don't you sit down and let us check your blood pressure?*

b) *Mr. Jones, you can let us take your pulse and blood pressure, ca<u>n't</u> you?*

Here is another example:

a) *Mr. Taylor, why don't you let us check you out and if you are medically okay, then we will leave.*

b) *Mr. Taylor, why don't you allow us to check you out and if you are medically okay we can leave. That's what you want isn't it?*

As you can see in both of these examples, the provider's approach is one that allows the patient to choose and answer with an affirmative response. When the patient is giving a positive response, they have been taken out of the defensive or aggressive mode and are instead placed into a cooperative mode. Once a cooperative mode is set, the patient will likely continue to cooperate with the provider. The provider has de-escalated the situation without the patient realizing what the provider has done.

Avoid Cornering the Patient

Cornering is the term we use to define steps that are mistakenly taken, either consciously or subconsciously, to gain control over the patient. Too often, when patients feel that someone is trying to gain control over them, they have only one recourse to maintain their independence . . . violence. To better understand the concept of cornering, we use the acronym CAPE. The acronym CAPE represents the four commonly used types of cornering techniques.

C—Contact Cornering

Contact cornering takes place when person-to-person contact is made. Oftentimes, the provider may contact corner a person without ever realizing it. To the verbally threatening patient, a gesture as simple as a hand on the shoulder may in fact make them feel cornered. The provider must be aware that any form of physical contact may make the patient feel cornered. In these cases the patient will normally respond in a physical mode of self-defense (see Figure 6-2).

A—Angulated Cornering

When we corner a person by angulation, we literally back them into a corner. Think of a docile, gentle animal. Normally, the animal will let you pet it and befriend it. Take the same animal, however, and back it into a corner. When the animal feels trapped in the corner, it feels it has no way out of the corner other than by overpowering you. The verbally threatening patient is no different. When we back them into a corner, the only way they can physically escape is to overpower us. The provider must be aware of the concept of angulated cornering and make certain that they avoid this form of cornering (see Figure 6-3).

P—Psychological Cornering

We psychologically corner a patient when we make the patient feel that they have one of two choices—either submit to our demands or attack and escape. Of the various forms of cornering, psychological cornering is the one that is most mistakenly made. The best way to avoid psychologically cornering your patient is to provide choices and allow them to make choices that are right for them. The provider can guide the patient through effective choice making. The significant difference is that the patient must be allowed to choose the right option in such a way that he or she feels they made the choice on their own (see Figure 6-4).

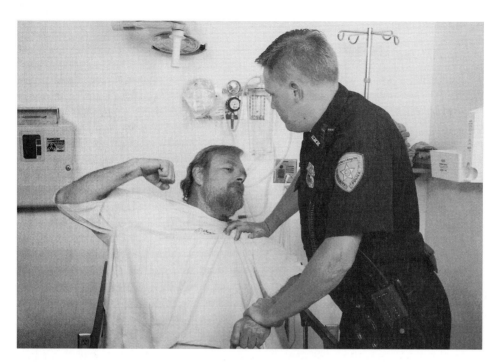

Figure 6-2 *This hospital security officer has contact cornered the patient by making physical contact. The patient can now be expected to react in a self-defense mode.*

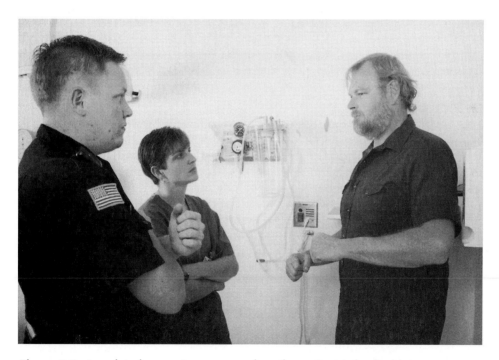

Figure 6-3 *Angulated cornering occurs when the patient is backed into a corner. Now the only way the patient can get out of the corner is by fighting.*

Figure 6-4 *Notice how the nurse and the security officer tower over the patient while talking down to him. This patient has been psychologically cornered.*

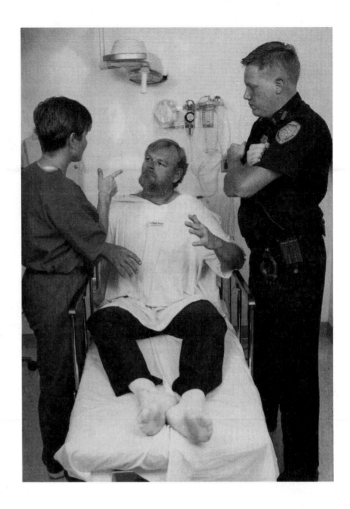

E—Exit Cornering

Exit cornering is another mistake that we often make without realizing it. When we exit corner a person, we physically place ourselves between them and the exit. Then the patient feels that the only way out of the exit is to go over the person who is blocking it. This is a common mistake made in treatment rooms of emergency departments, when a nurse or physician positions themselves between a patient and the door. Unfortunately, well-intentioned prehospital providers also make the same mistake in the field. Whether the patient has the option of leaving or not, the provider can avoid exit cornering by simply standing off to the side of the exit. This leaves the patient feeling that the exit is unblocked and accessible (see Figure 6-5).

Anticipate Violence

We have already established that when a patient is in this fourth step he or she is one step away from a physical form of aggression. The providers must realize this and begin preparing themselves for a possible physical attack. While there is still one critical step left between verbal threats and physical violence, the provider must begin to think of self-defense and self-preservation. It is at this point that the provider may consider withdrawing and calling for additional assistance.

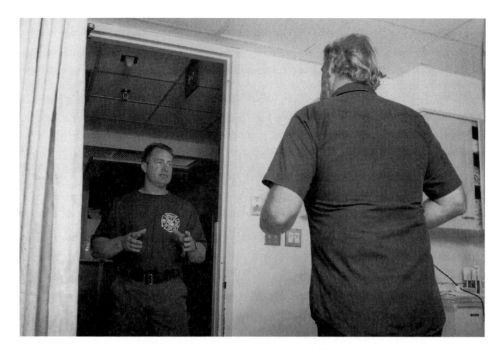

Figure 6-5 *Exit cornering occurs when the provider is physically between the patient and the exit. The patient feels he has but one way out—to overpower the provider.*

Physically Threatening Behavior

When a patient becomes physically threatening, the prehospital provider must be prepared for violence. If withdrawal is an option, it should be given serious consideration. If de-escalation attempts are going to continue, the prehospital provider must consider the following:

Recognize the Critical Point

When the patient becomes physically threatening, the provider must realize that they have, for all intent and purposes, lost control of the situation. Often the patient's body language begins to dictate to the provider what is going to happen next. In many cases the patient may take a physical stance that suggests impending physical violence. The patient may also begin to scan the room or the environment looking for objects that could be used as a weapon against the provider or others in the room. *If withdrawal is an option, this is the last chance to exercise it.*

Maintain a Defensive Posture

The provider must continue to be cognizant of his or her body language. Earlier in this chapter we discussed the initial interview position. One of the key benefits of this position is that it allows the provider to change from the nonthreatening stance to a defensive stance, often unnoticed by the patient. To do so, the provider simply moves his right foot back one step and turns it at a 45-degree angle. In doing so, the provider has improved his or her physical balance and is now ready to defend against a physical attack. Just as in the initial interview position, the hands are kept at chest height, where they can be seen by the patient. This still conveys to the patient that the provider holds no weapons and allows the provider to have his or her hands readily available should it be necessary to physically block an attack by the patient (see Figure 6-6).

Look for Strong-Side and Weak-Side Indicators

Most people have a strong side and a weak side. Some studies suggest that up to 93% of people are right handed; the right side is their strong side. The well-prepared provider can observe a patient and normally be able to identify strong side and weak side indicators.

Listed below are some common indicators that the provider can use to identify the patient's strong side and weak side. It must be noted that *these are not always 100% reliable; instead, they are provided as a guideline for the provider to use so that he or she may physically position themselves appropriately* (see Figure 6-7).

Strong-Side/Weak-Side Indicators

- Most men part their hair on the weak side.
- Most men wear their watch on the weak side.
- Most men put on their belt in such a way that the tip of the belt points to the weak side. Women's belts often point to the strong side.
- Most men carry their wallets on the strong side.
- Most men carry pens, cigarettes, or lighters in a weak-side shirt pocket.

Figure 6-6 *From the initial interview position, the prehospital provider can easily change to a defensive stance, which offers improved balance and greater personal safety.*

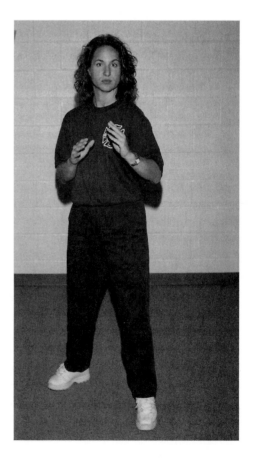

Chapter 6: Defusing Aggressive Behavior

- Most men will carry pens, checkbooks, and other like items on the weak side of sport coats or suit coats.
- Most women will carry their purse on their strong side.
- Most people will stand with their strong-side leg slightly bent.
- Most people will stand with the weak-side shoulder slightly dipped.
- Most people will carry a pager or cellular phone on their strong side.
- Most people will carry keys in a strong-side pocket.

If the provider is able to identify strong-side and weak-side indicators, they can then position themselves on the patient's weak side. If a patient is going to attack, and avoidance does not seem possible, it is preferable that the provider be positioned on the person's weak side. This is true not only because of the difference in strength between the strong side and the weak side, but also in the difference of coordination as well. If a person attacks from their weak side, there is a greater chance that the provider will be able to physically subdue the person than if the person is attacking from their strong side. Additionally, since most people attack with their strong side, if the provider is positioned on the weak side of the patient, the patient will have a greater distance to cover to attack the provider, giving the provider additional time to prepare to defend him- or herself.

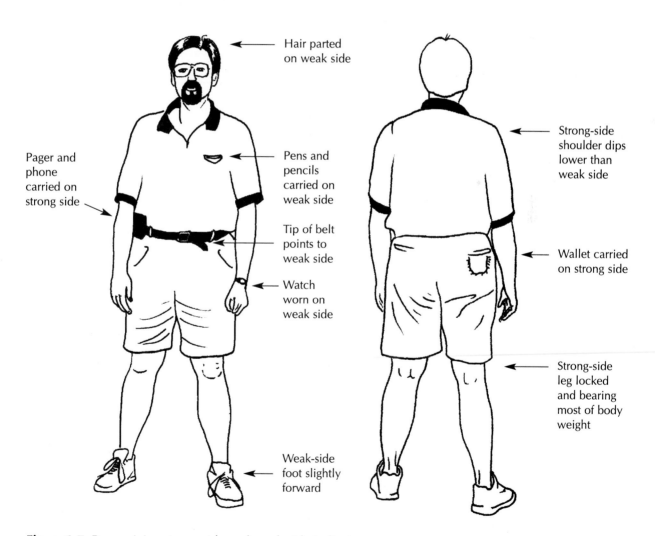

Figure 6-7 *Recognizing strong-side and weak-side indicators.*

Be Prepared for a Physical Attack

Again, it cannot be overemphasized that whenever possible *withdrawal is the option of choice.* If the provider can leave the area, this is the best option. If for some reason the provider cannot leave, then he or she must be prepared for a physical attack.

Even if a physical attack occurs, the provider must continue to act in a prudent and professional manner. When an attack occurs, the provider must focus on self-preservation and self-defense but must still remain focused on the needs of the patient. Self-preservation and self-defense are not about fighting or injuring the patient. Instead, the provider wants to prevent injury from occurring to themselves and to their patient. The purpose of training in techniques of self-defense is to prevent injury to oneself and to regain control of the patient. It is not about fighting with the patient.

The provider must also recognize that they are accountable for their actions. If, in the course of dealing with a physically aggressive patient, the provider should injure the patient, the provider will still be held accountable for his or her actions. Providers are only human. When someone is attacking us, it is easy for our fight or flight system to take over and our adrenaline to kick in. Once the provider gains control of the patient, he or she must refocus their energy on keeping the patient under control in the manner least harmful to the patient.

Physically Violent Behavior

When a patient becomes physically violent toward the provider, the provider must be prepared to transfer from a *talk down mode* to a *takedown mode.*

Takedown is the process by which control of the patient is regained, and the patient is subdued in such a manner that he or she can be restrained from hurting themselves and others. Chapters 7 and 8 will address in more depth the physical side of aggression management.

Nonverbal Clues of Impending Physical Violence

During the entire time that the provider is dealing with the patient, he or she must always be aware of nonverbal clues indicating that trouble is imminent. By watching out for some of the following nonverbal clues, the provider will often have insight into what the patient is going to do and can take a pro-active instead of reactive approach.

Some nonverbal clues that the patient may demonstrate include the following:

Sudden Movements to the Prehospital Provider
The patient may make sudden moves toward the provider as a bluff tactic. In doing so, the patient is assessing the provider's preparedness for a physical attack. If the provider seems unprepared, there is greater likelihood that the patient may attack. The provider who is prepared stands less chance of being physically attacked.

Tightening of Small and Large Muscle Groups
The patient may begin to tighten or flex different muscle groups as a sign of power or strength or in an attempt to intimidate the provider. Oftentimes

the twitching will be done in such a way that the provider is able to recognize the dominant side of the aggressor and can be prepared for an attack from that side.

Twitching of Facial Muscles
Twitching of facial muscles can be an indication of stress, anxiety, or apprehension. Uncontrolled twitching is often a precipitating sign of physical violence.

Darting Eye Movements
Darting eye movements are another valuable nonverbal clue and often indicate that the aggressor is uncertain of his next move, may be looking for an exit, or may be preparing to make a fast, sudden move.

Fixed Staring
Fixed staring can be an attempt at intimidation or it may indicate an impending attack. The provider will not want to get into a staring contest with an aggressive patient, however, it is important to maintain eye contact. If the provider is being stared down, avoiding eye contact will send a signal to the aggressor that he is in fact intimidating the provider.

Glancing for Weapons
If the aggressor starts to scan the surrounding environment, the provider must be on the alert for what the aggressor might be looking for. The provider must be aware of any nearby articles that the aggressor could pick up and use as a weapon.

Shifting Balance
Constantly shifting one's balance is often a sign of nervousness or apprehension. It may also be an attempt by the aggressor to gain a position from which it is physically comfortable for him or her to lunge or attack.

Raised Voice Pitch and Increased Volume
As the aggressor becomes more agitated, you may notice distinct changes in the pitch or volume of his or her voice. This is another indication that the individual is moving up the continuum and that your de-escalation efforts are not successful. Changes in voice pitch or volume are a sign of increasing stress and anxiety.

Increased Breathing Rate
An increase in breathing rate indicates stress and anxiety in the individual. The more stressed and apprehensive the individual, the more his or her breathing rate will increase.

All these nonverbal clues, either individually or in any combination, should indicate to the provider potential changes in the patient's behaviors, which may lead to physical violence. The provider must be watching for these changes and consider the best tactical approach.

Some Do's and Don'ts of Aggression Management

There are some simple do's and don'ts that the provider can practice to increase the likelihood of successful verbal de-escalation. First, lets look at the don't list:

1. Don't give the patient orders instead of choices.
2. Don't project an "I don't give a damn" attitude.
3. Don't over stare the patient.
4. Don't make threats toward the patient.

5. Don't argue or offer compromises to the patient.
6. Don't become emotionally attached.
7. Don't corner the patient.
8. Don't violate your patient's space.
9. Don't lie to the patient.
10. Don't turn your back on the patient.

In addition to these don'ts, there is also a list of things on the do list that the provider must keep in mind:

1. Do monitor your own status.
2. Do allow someone else to take over de-escalation attempts if you become angry, frustrated, or fearful.
3. Do demonstrate self-confidence.
4. Do stay calm and relaxed.
5. Do keep voice pitch and voice volume down.
6. Do allow the patient to make choices.
7. Do offer honest options and choices.
8. Do allow the patient to save self-esteem.
9. Do maintain a safe personal distance.
10. DO TAKE YOUR TIME.

Summary

In Chapter 4 and again in this chapter we have looked at the aggression continuum repeatedly. The healthcare provider must be able to observe behaviors demonstrated by the patient and place that behavior appropriately on the aggression continuum. Once the provider has placed the behavior at the appropriate level on the continuum, he or she must then be able to equate the behavior level with the appropriate de-escalation techniques.

De-escalation takes time. The provider must be prepared to take as much time as necessary to bring the situation to a state of calm. The provider must always realize that a state of calm will always be restored. Successful de-escalation is based upon the techniques that are used to restore the state of calm. The importance of recognizing when one is in danger of personal injury or attack and the importance of backing out when safely able to do so cannot be overstressed. Assistance from additional police, fire, security, or other providers should always be readily available whenever de-escalating a potentially aggressive situation. To go into a potentially violent situation without adequate backup available is not only ludicrous, but may also be suicidal.

Escapes from Grabs and Holds

Here Comes the Bride . . .

Jennifer Mobeley was walking on clouds. As a paramedic, she routinely had the opportunity to help other people. She had graduated at the top of her class a year earlier and had already received an award for valor after saving two children from a burning car before the fire department arrived. Now, after dating Jeff McNeil for the past two years, she was two days away from becoming his wife. Things could not be better.

The previous day had been wonderful. Jenny's mother and sister joined her for the final fitting of her wedding dress. Since she was a little girl, Jenny had dreamed of a Victorian-era wedding dress, and now a dressmaker was making one especially for her. It was a two-piece dress with a bustle and train made of ivory ribbed silk. The dressmaker enhanced the dress with banded silk-plush panels on the skirt and ruched tulle at the neck and wrists. When Jenny first saw it, she could not contain her tears of joy. Even as a little girl, she had never dreamed of such a beautiful dress. Jenny opted against a traditional veil, however. Instead, she chose to have her long auburn hair permed into flowing textured locks, her natural hair color complementing the fall flowers she would carry. Everything seemed to be falling into place; her dream was coming true.

The shift had been quiet, as Jenny hoped. For the first time in her career, her focus was on something other than her job. All she wanted to do now was to get through the shift and be one day closer to becoming Mrs. Jeff McNeil.

As she finished putting the dinner dishes back in the cabinet, her thoughts again wandered to what she envisioned her wedding day to be like. Sunny. Cool. Blue skies. Organ music. Family. Friends. What could break the dream?

The ringing of the alarm broke her dream. "Ambulance 1441, a possible overdose at 12203 Clayborn Drive. Caller advises that her baby has swallowed a bottle of pills. Caller requests no lights and siren. No further information available. Time of dispatch is 2008 hours."

En route, Jenny was quiet. Her thoughts were still not focused on the response, instead running last-minute tasks through her mind. As the ambulance parked in the driveway, Jenny grabbed the pediatric jump bag and started into the house. A middle-aged woman met her hysterically at the door and directed her to an upstairs bedroom. As Jenny entered the bedroom, she sensed something was wrong—this did not appear to be a baby's room. Before she could react, Jenny suddenly felt a painful pressure on her head and quickly realized that someone had grabbed her by her hair.

She tried to scream but fear prevented her from making a sound. Where was her partner, she wondered. What was going on here?

"Jenny . . . be careful," the voice of her partner called from the stairs. "The baby is 28 years old and may get violent . . ."

In her frozen fear, Jenny thought of the aggression management and self-defense class the company had sponsored for continuing education recently. She had opted not to attend, figuring her charm and femininity would allow her to talk her way out of anything. Now, in a moment of fear and pain, she could make no sound.

The patient started to drag her farther into the bedroom by her hair. She remembered the guys on the previous shift talking about how to escape a hair grab. What did they say . . . how did that work . . . what should she do? She heard his sadistic laughter and knew she had to get free quickly. The pain of her hair being pulled was causing her to become dizzy . . . he obviously had large hands and was holding a great deal of her hair. Not knowing what else to do, Jenny did the worse thing she could do . . . she pulled back against his hand. As she did, she felt the tearing sensation in her head and then suddenly she was free. Startled, she looked up and saw the man . . . a small man . . . a glazed and confused look in his eyes. What she saw in his hand was unmistakable . . . her hair. A large mat of her hair from the top of her head.

Jenny reached up and felt the unimaginable . . . a large clump of her beautiful hair had been pulled out of her head, leaving a painful bald spot in its place. As her partner and police arrived on the scene, Jenny staggered out of the room. She was injured but more shocked. All she could imagine now was walking down the aisle in two days, being stared at by everyone.

The most important day of her life had just been taken from her.

• • • • • • • • • •

Where did Jenny go wrong? Did the outcome have to be so catastrophic for the young bride-to-be? Obviously not, but like so many healthcare providers, Jenny failed to prepare for the physical encounters that victimized her.

In this chapter, we will look at some of the common grabs and holds used against healthcare workers. In addition, we will introduce and discuss techniques to minimize injuries to the prehospital provider as well as to the patient.

Introduction

This chapter is designed to acquaint the healthcare provider with basic information on how to safely approach patients while respecting their personal space. In addition, you will learn basic escapes from the common grabs and holds encountered on the street. *It is highly recommended that providers attend a training course conducted by a competent instructor who specializes in self-defense. In no way should this chapter be construed as a stand-alone training program. It is important for you to remember that this chapter is based on your right to defend yourself. The techniques are not to be used in an offensive manner.* You are responsible for knowing the laws in your state in addition to your applicable department or organizational policy before using any type of force.

Before approaching any situation, you should ask yourself: Do I need assistance? Assistance may be additional providers, police, security, or any other potential support staff. Know in advance where to obtain proper assistance, and do not hesitate to request it. It is better to request assistance and not need it than to need it and not request it. Many providers injured in the line of duty will tell you that they sensed danger but felt they could handle the situation. Human beings have instincts to keep them away from dangerous situations. Unfortunately, our instincts often take a back seat to our desire to help. If your instincts tell you there is danger, trust them.

Approaching the Patient

Many healthcare providers are injured during their approach to a patient, even when the patient has not exhibited any signs of unruliness. Although the provider is approaching with the best of intentions, patients may construe the provider's approach as an act of aggression and may lash out at this point. If your approach is done safely, you lessen the risk of becoming a victim. The following steps should be considered in every approach to a patient, even if the patient has no history of violence.

1. **Always begin talking to the patient from a safe distance.** Let the patient know you are there to help. The way in which the patient reacts to your voice oftentimes will indicate whether you should anticipate violence.

2. **As you approach the patient, begin assessing the environment.** How many people are present? Do they appear friendly or hostile? Is this a crime scene? Are there weapons present? Weapons, of course, include the obvious—knives and guns—but also the not-so obvious. For example, one of the most common weapons used in domestic violence is an ordinary table fork. What other common household objects might be used as weapons? Pencils, pens, pots and pans, boards, hot beverages, rope, tools, glassware, lamps, fireplace tools, and heavy blunt instruments are often overlooked as potential weapons (see Figure 7-1). In the hospital, the same applies. Think of all the common instruments and equipment that can be used as weapons. Stethoscopes, scissors, scalpels, bedpans, and IV poles have all been used as weapons against healthcare providers. The list is virtually endless, and it's usually the item you didn't think about that gets used against you.

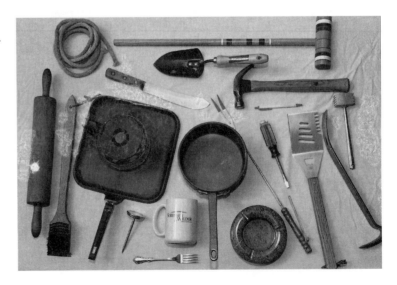

Figure 7-1 _Prehospital providers must always be aware of the common household items that can become deadly when used as weapons._

Personal Space Zone

Each of us has an invisible barrier around us that we do not like invaded, especially by strangers. The length or size of the "zone" differs between individuals, but in a confrontational situation, the size of the zone generally increases. Trial after trial reveals that the zone also varies depending on the direction of the approach. As someone approaches from the front, most of us will start to get an uneasy feeling at approximately three feet. As someone approaches from either side, we begin to feel uncomfortable when the person enters our peripheral vision. From the rear, we get uncomfortable as soon as we know the person is there and will usually maneuver ourselves into a position to completely avoid the rear approach. Although you cannot properly assess and treat a patient unless you are within their personal space, it is still important for you to respect the patient's zone and be aware that there is an increased risk of violence when entering this space.

There are some simple precautions you can take to minimize your risk when entering a patient's personal space. First, tell the patient what you are doing and why you are doing it and solicit their cooperation. For example: "Mr. Jensen, I need to place an oxygen mask over your mouth and nose to help your breathing. Is that okay?" This simple procedure lets the patient know you're not trying to hurt him and asks his permission. The patient feels in control and is not threatened. On the other hand, if the patient tells you to stay away, you now have an indication that this may become a violent situation and you may need additional help.

Even if you now have the patient's permission to assist him or her, approach with caution. Keep in mind that every patient, regardless of age, sex, or size, has the potential to harm you. By following some basic steps during every approach, you can again minimize the risk of serious injury. As you approach a patient, watch and listen for any sudden changes in their demeanor. Keep your hands in front of your body at approximately chest level (see Figure 7-2). If a patient strikes out, your hands will be in a position to block their strike and protect yourself (see Figure 7-3). Maintain a proper balance. Keep your feet approximately a shoulder width apart, your knees slightly bent, and your weight evenly divided between both legs. Again, remember to talk to your patients to make them feel at ease. Let them know what you are doing so that you're not adding to their fear. While this may seem routine to you, it probably isn't to your patient.

Escaping Grabs and Holds

Unfortunately, with all of our best efforts, there will still be situations in which the patient will try to grab, punch, kick, or bite. The remainder of this chapter focuses on how to escape from grabs, holds, and bites, while the next chapter focuses on punches and kicks.

For the purpose of this text, we will address the more common types of grabs, holds, and bites, including wrist grabs and handshake holds, hair grabs, clothing grabs, chokeholds, headlocks, and various bites. Keep in mind, though, that every situation is different. Attacks happen when you least expect them, and there are as many different types of attacks as there are people. In addition, the techniques described are not the only ones available and may have to be adjusted according to the situation.

Figure 7-2 *Always remember to convey a nonthreatening posture so the patient doesn't feel that he must defend himself against you.*

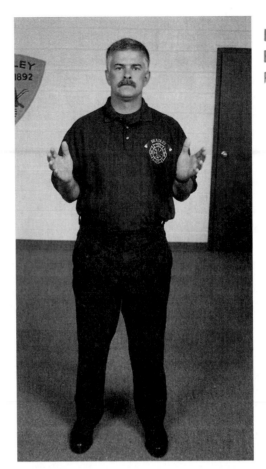

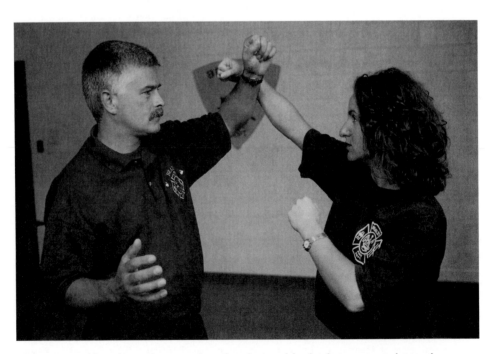

Figure 7-3 *If hands are kept at chest level, a suddenly thrown punch can be blocked and the prehospital provider can defend himself from further attack.*

The more you learn and practice the techniques, the more confident you'll become in their application and use.

Wrist Grabs and Handshake Hold

One-Hand Wrist Grab

When someone grabs you by the wrist, most people will react by pulling away, often causing more injury. Instead, step back slightly to bring *him or her* off balance; you can then break free by turning your wrist and pulling away *at the point where his or her thumb is around the wrist* (see Figure 7-4). The thumb is the weakest part of the hold and most people, despite size or strength, can free themselves in this manner. Remember to call for assistance and maneuver yourself into a better position should your aggressor continue toward you.

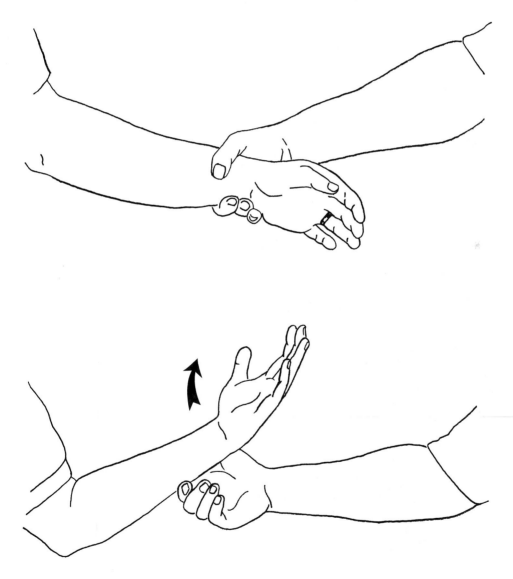

Figure 7-4 *One-hand wrist escape.*

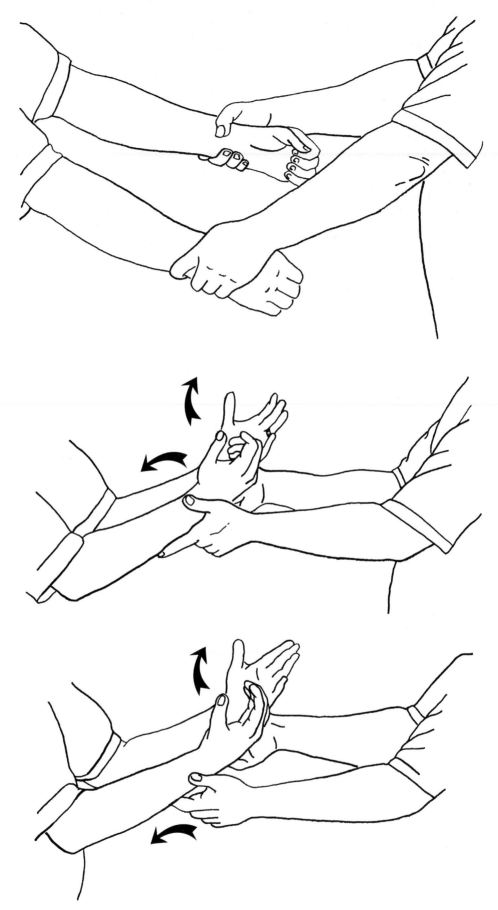

Figure 7-5 *Two-hand wrist escape.*

Two-Hand Wrist Grab

If you are grabbed by both wrists, you may use the same maneuver applied in the one-hand wrist grab. Again, step back slightly to bring the aggressor off balance, then turn your wrist and pull away at the point where their thumb is around your wrist (see Figure 7-5). Remember to call for assistance and maneuver yourself into a better position should your aggressor continue toward you.

Handshake Hold

Many times, aggressors will appear friendly and even put out their hand "in friendship" to deceive you. The best rule of thumb is not to shake hands with people you don't know and trust. However, should you get yourself into a situation in which someone has you in a powerful hand-shake and won't let you out, simply place your free hand over his or her thumb and pull it away from your hand. This will loosen their grip, allowing you to work yourself free (see Figure 7-6). Remember to call for assistance and maneuver yourself into a better position should your aggressor continue toward you.

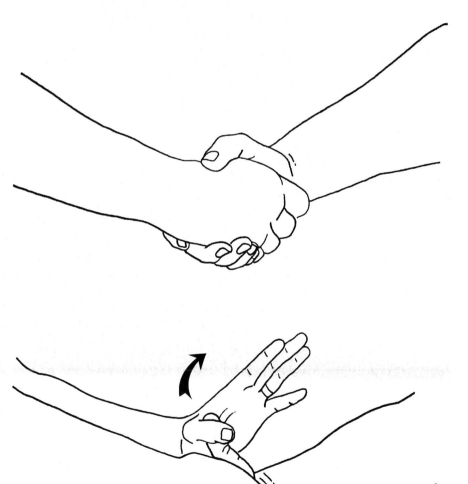

Figure 7-6 *Escape from handshake hold.*

Front Hair Grab

The normal reaction to being grabbed by the hair is to jerk away. Jerking away can cause severe pain and discomfort, not to mention hair loss. However, *if someone places you in a front hair grab, immediately put both of your hands over the aggressor's hand to trap it tightly to your head.* This maneuver will keep the aggressor from being able to pull out your hair (see Figure 7-7a). Next, take a step back to take the aggressor off balance, then turn your body, placing your elbow against the aggressor's elbow and

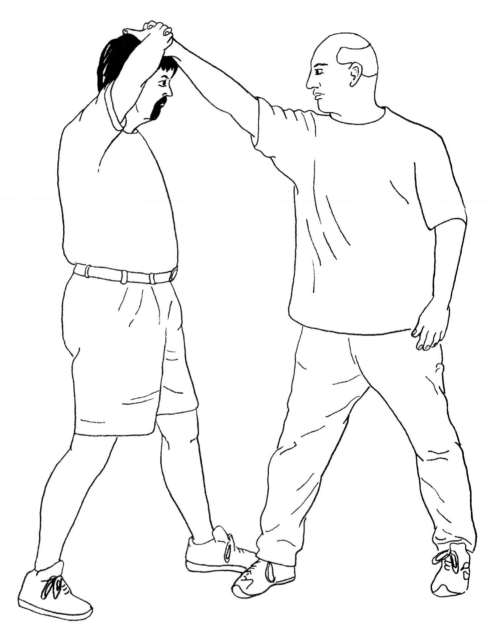

Figure 7-7a *Escape from front hair grab. With the aggressor's hand trapped, he cannot pull away. You have taken control of his action. Then step back to take the aggressor off balance.*

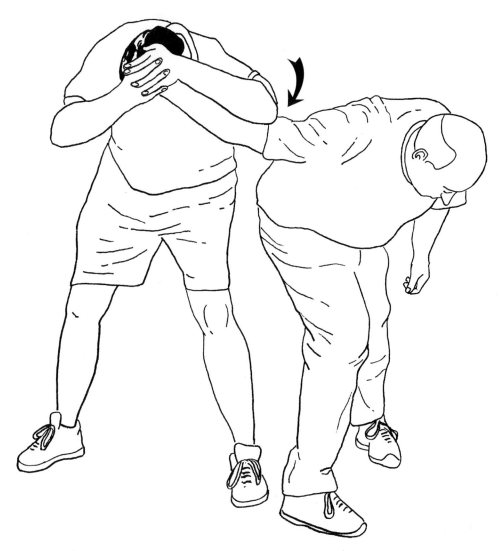

Figure 7-7b *Escape from front hair grab. The aggressor's arm is now locked at the elbow by your elbow. In this position, a person of average strength can take the aggressor down.*

continue turning into the elbow and downward until the aggressor loses his or her grip (see Figure 7-7b). It is important to note that locking a person's elbow puts them in a position in which they cannot defy your control. This is a key maneuver that, with minimal force, allows the provider to escape this and other grabs. Remember to call for assistance and maneuver yourself into a better position should your aggressor continue toward you.

Rear Hair Grab

If someone grabs your hair from the rear, *avoid the reaction to pull away.* Place both of your hands over the aggressor's hand to trap it tightly to your head. Next, take a step *forward* to take the aggressor off balance, then turn your body into the aggressor's elbow and continue turning into the elbow and downward until the aggressor loses his or her grip (see Figures 7-8a and 7-8b). Remember to call for assistance and maneuver yourself into a better position should your aggressor continue toward you.

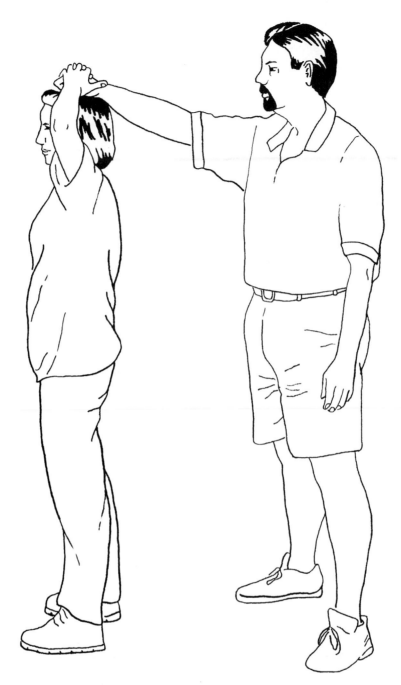

Figure 7-8a *Escape from rear hair grab. Trap the aggressor's hand to your head. You have taken control of his action.*

Clothing Grab

Aggressors will often grab your shirt at the lapel in an attempt to intimidate you. Once again, resist the urge to pull away. Instead, place one hand over the aggressor's hand, locking it in place (see Figure 7-9a). Take your free hand and distract the aggressor by pinching the underside of their arm, slapping toward their eyes, or by shouting in a distinct tone (see Figure 7-9b). Simultaneously, peel the offender's hand away from your

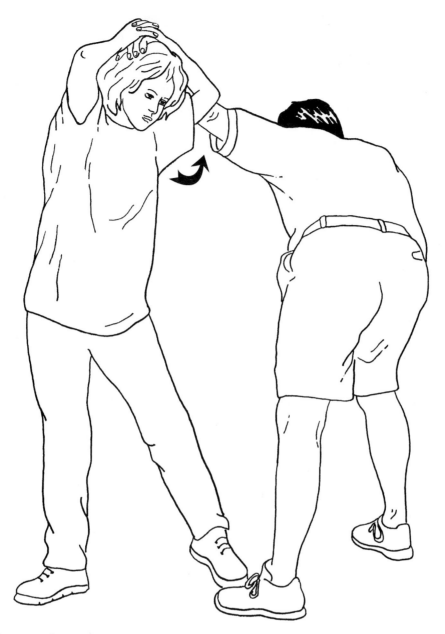

Figure 7-8b _Escape from rear hair grab. Lock the aggressor's arm with your elbow to take him down._

shirt, turning their wrist in an inward or outward motion. Use your free hand to lock the aggressor's arm at his elbow and force him down until he lets go (see Figure 7-9c). Remember to call for assistance and maneuver yourself into a better position should your aggressor continue toward you.

Another common clothing grab is one in which the aggressor puts their hand against your chest, with their palm in, and grabs your shirt. Immediately place both your hands over the aggressor's hand to trap it in place, then bend at the waist toward the aggressor and downward until the aggressor goes down to the ground. Remember to call for assistance and maneuver yourself into a better position should your aggressor continue toward you.

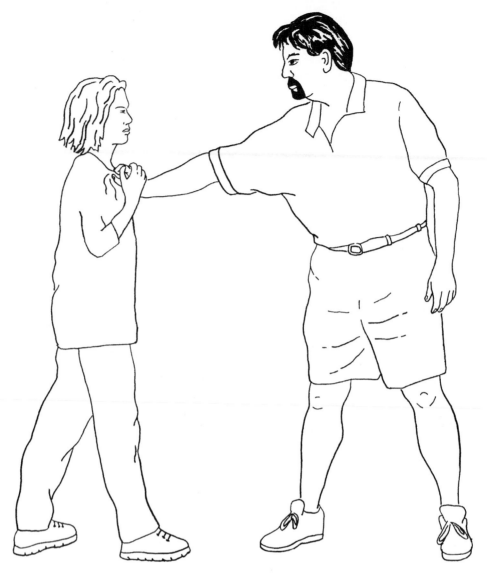

Figure 7-9a *Escape from clothing grab. Trap the aggressor's hand to take control of his action.*

Figure 7-9b *Escape from clothing grab. With your free hand, distract the aggressor by pinching his arm.*

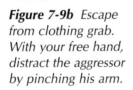

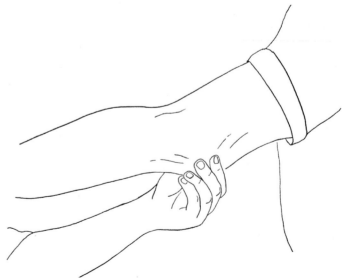

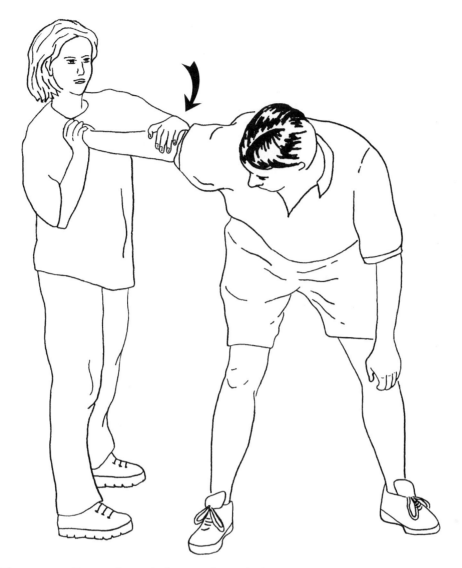

Figure 7-9c *Escape from clothing grab. Lock the aggressor's arm at his elbow and take him down.*

Healthcare providers can do some pre-planning to minimize the chances of getting hurt during a clothing grab. First, try not to wear clothing that is extremely loose. Much the same as the factory worker knows not to wear loose clothing around machinery, the healthcare provider should also realize that wearing loose clothing can be an occupational hazard. Loose clothing is easier to grab, twist, and hold. Second, never wear jewelry, stethoscopes, ties, scarves, or other articles around your neck because these could be grabbed and used to strangle you. If you must wear a necklace, take it to your jeweler and have them put a breakaway link in it. If you must wear a tie, make sure it is the clip-on or breakaway type to avoid getting choked with it. Stethoscopes can be dangerous for a variety of reasons. If worn around the neck, they can be grabbed on both sides and used to choke the caregiver. If the stethoscope is pulled away from the neck, it can easily be used as a whipping weapon. With that in mind, you may want to carry your stethoscope in your pocket.

Front Chokehold

The Inverted V Technique

There are numerous ways to defeat a front chokehold. The important thing to remember is that you must act quickly. *It only takes three to five seconds for a properly applied chokehold to render you unconscious.* One move that is not difficult to apply and is easy to remember is the inverted V technique. This technique is accomplished by placing both of your hands together with your elbows out in an inverted V shape, under the aggressor's arms. Then drive your arms upward, with as much force as you can generate, between the aggressor's arms to break the chokehold (see Figure 7-10).

Techniques to Avoid the Front Chokehold

A one-hand grab from the front is when the aggressor reaches out for the caregiver with one arm in an attempt to grab the throat. Whichever hand the aggressor is reaching with, take a side step in the same direction, raise your arm on the same side you are stepping in and redirect the aggressor's hand away from your throat before he can grab it. Keep your other hand up to protect yourself should the aggressor continue the attack.

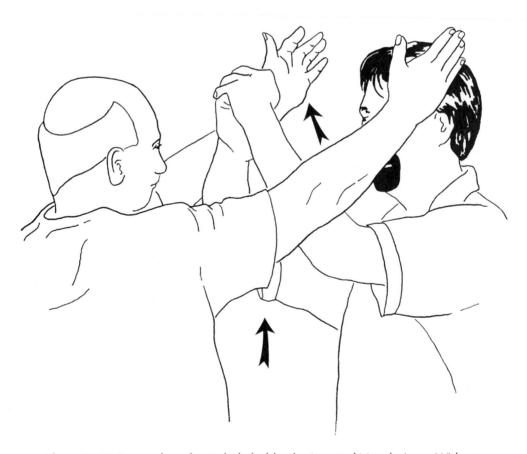

Figure 7-10 *Escape from front chokehold—the inverted V technique. With your arms in an inverted V shape, rapidly force them up between the aggressor's arms to release his chokehold.*

A two-hand grab from the front is where the aggressor reaches out with both hands for the caregiver in an attempt to grab the throat. This time take a step toward either side and raise your arm on that same side to redirect the aggressor's arms away from your throat. Once again, keep your other arm up and ready should the aggressor continue the attack.

The Front Windmill Technique

The front windmill technique is a very effective way to escape a two-hand chokehold and is performed by simply raising one arm and rotating your body across the front of the offender's body, bringing your extended arm down across his in a motion similar to the blades of a windmill (see Figures 7-11a and 7-11b).

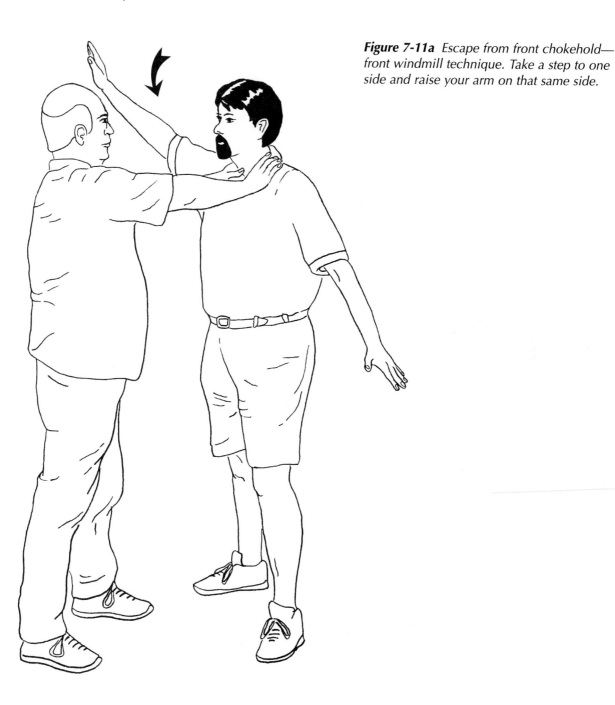

Figure 7-11a *Escape from front chokehold— front windmill technique. Take a step to one side and raise your arm on that same side.*

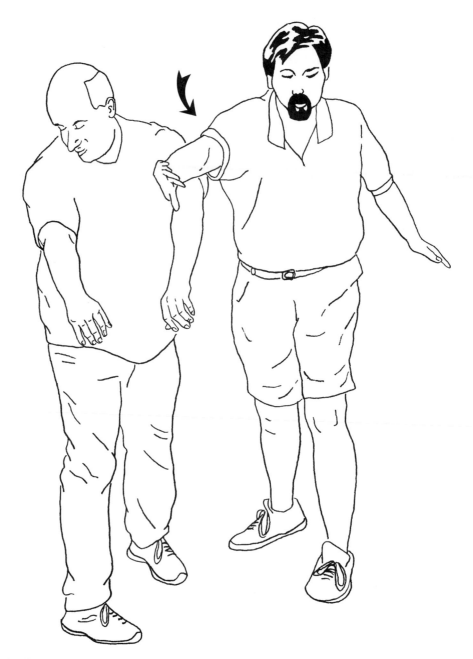

Figure 7-11b *Escape from front chokehold—front windmill technique. Rotate your extended arm down across the aggressor's arms in a motion similar to the blades of a windmill.*

Rear Chokehold

The Reverse Windmill Technique

In defending against a chokehold from the rear, the technique used to keep yourself from getting into a rear chokehold depends on how the aggressor attempts to grab you. If the aggressor attempts to place his or her hands around your throat, you can easily apply the reverse windmill technique. This technique is accomplished by raising one arm over your body and quickly turning to the rear on the same side as the raised arm. Continue spinning your body and the leading arm to the rear, into the aggressor's arm to prevent him from grabbing your throat. If the aggressor *has already* placed his or her hands around your throat, you can easily apply the reverse windmill technique described to break his chokehold (see Figures 7-12a and 7-12b). Remember to call for assistance and maneuver yourself into a better position should your aggressor continue toward you.

Another common chokehold from the rear is when the aggressor places his or her arm over your head and around your throat, holding you between their forearm and biceps. *This type of chokehold is extremely dangerous and life threatening, demanding immediate reaction on your part.* Unfortunately, since this hold is applied from the rear, you may not be

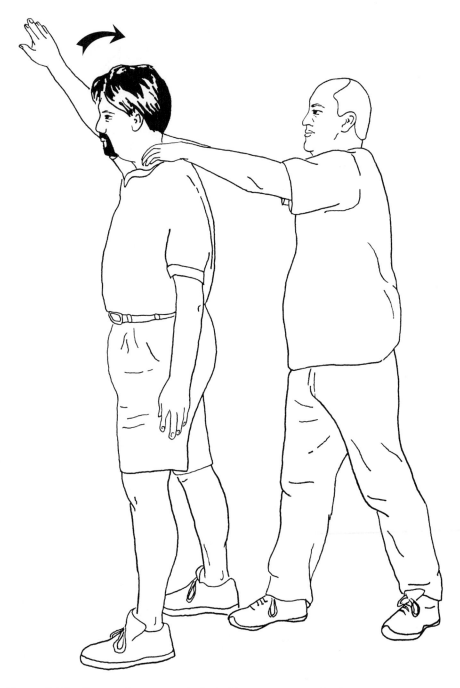

Figure 7-12a *Escape from rear chokehold—reverse windmill technique. Extend one arm to start your windmill motion.*

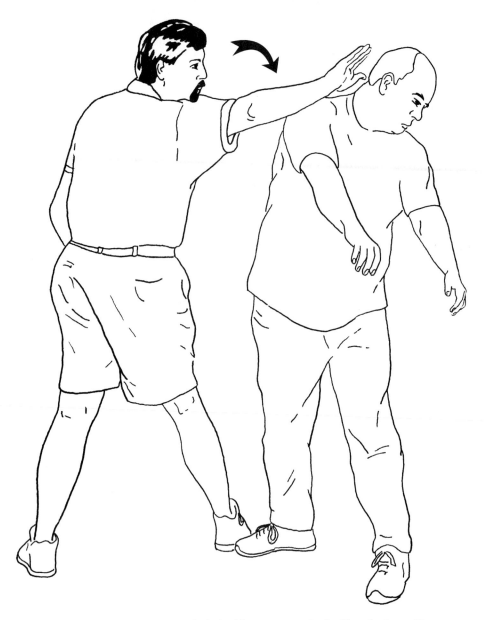

Figure 7-12b *Escape from rear chokehold—reverse windmill technique. Keep your arm extended, turn on the same side as your extended arm toward the aggressor, and rotate your arm against his in a motion similar to blades of a windmill.*

able to block the attack. If you see the attack coming, simply tuck your chin, grab the aggressors arm, and raise the arm straight up while lowering your own body to avoid the choke. If you are unable to avoid the choke, at the moment you feel the aggressor's arm around your neck, reach up with both hands and grab it to prevent him or her from choking you to the point of unconsciousness. Immediately tuck your chin and turn your head toward the aggressor's elbow. While holding the aggressor's arm, raise one of your feet approximately one foot off the ground. Turn the raised foot outward and move it back until you feel it touch the aggressor's leg. When it does, immediately rake your foot down the aggressors leg and shin, exerting as much force as possible on the aggressor's instep. (It takes approximately seven pounds of pressure to break the instep.)

When the aggressor loosens his or her grip, break yourself free, call for assistance, and get yourself into a better position should the aggressor continue the attack.

Headlock

If someone gets you into a headlock, immediately tuck your chin down and turn your head toward his or her elbow to avoid choking (see Figure 7-13a). With your arm closest to the aggressor's body, reach over the aggressor's head and place your finger under his or her nose. Begin applying

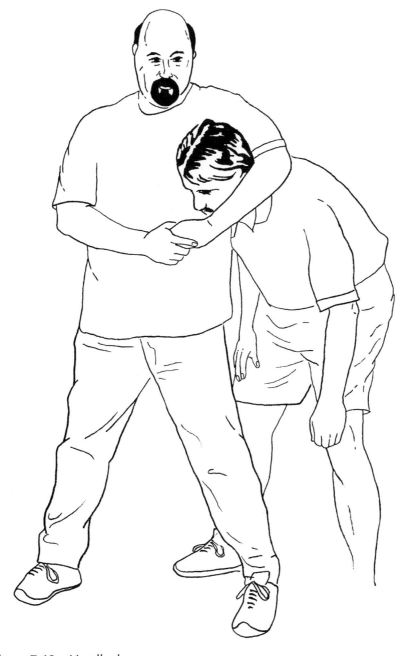

Figure 7-13a *Headlock escape.*

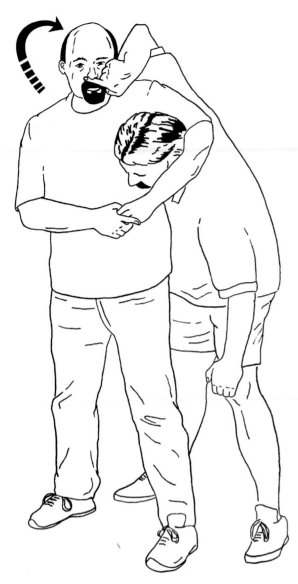

Figure 7-13b *Headlock escape. Bring your inside arm over the aggressor's shoulder and head and place your finger under his nose. Be sure to keep your chin down and your head tucked in to prevent from being choked.*

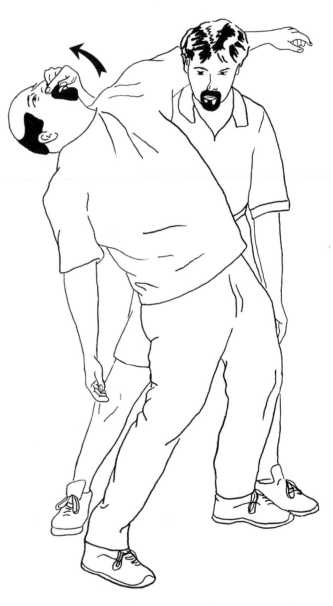

Figure 7-13c *Headlock escape. Apply pressure under the aggressor's nose, pushing toward the center of his head. He will quickly be brought off balance and will likely release you in the process.*

Chapter 7: Escapes from Grabs and Holds

upward pressure under their nose toward the center of their head (see Figure 7-13b). Continue to bring your arm backward causing the aggressor to bend backward until you are free (see Figure 7-13c). Remember to call for assistance and maneuver yourself into a better position should your aggressor continue toward you.

Bites

A human bite is one of the most painful and dangerous injuries you can encounter. Obviously, the best thing to do is avoid letting an aggressive patient get close enough to bite you. Unfortunately, it can and does happen. If an aggressor bites you, place a finger directly under their nose and apply rapid pressure upward at about a 45-degree angle toward the center of their head until they loosen their bite (see Figure 7-14). Remember to call for assistance and maneuver yourself into a better position should your aggressor continue toward you.

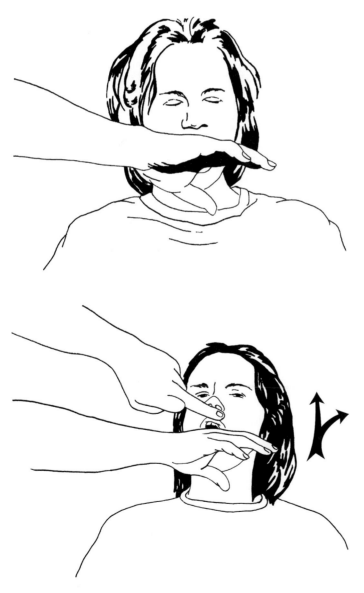

Figure 7-14 Escape from bite. Place your finger under the aggressor's nose and apply rapid pressure upward at a 45-degree angle toward the center of her head until she loosen her bite.

Summary

You do not need to take up martial arts to be an effective healthcare provider. You do, however, owe it to yourself and your loved ones to learn and practice basic assault prevention techniques. If you regularly practice and teach the techniques covered in this text, they will work for you. These techniques were chosen because they are simple to apply and easy to remember.

Self-defense techniques are only useful when someone is actually being attacked or assaulted. Such actions may be totally avoided by applying the methodology learned in Chapters 3, 4, 5, and 6. Pre-planning, recognition of potential violence, and team intervention will go a long way to defusing aggressive behavior before a physical confrontation. It is in everyone's best interest to avoid an altercation.

Realistically, however, violence may be inevitable regardless of the steps you take to avoid a physical altercation. As a result, these techniques were developed as a practical and effective way to respond in a critical and/or hostile situation.

Basic Blocking and Takedown Techniques

When Healthcare Professionals Must Use Force

Angie was a new graduate nurse, barely out of school. She was on duty on the Orthopedic Unit, 6 South, one night when the "seasoned" nurses were talking about the patient in room 614, Marvin Turner. None of them wanted to go into his room because he always shouted, cursed, and sometimes even grabbed them as they tried to work around him. And, of course, he was the one who kept the nurse call button in his hand around the clock. He actually slept with it. Angie, being a new grad, volunteered to take care of Turner. After all, she learned in school that patients will respond with respect if you treat them with dignity and respect. Besides, Angie had trained to the black-belt level in aikido, a form of martial arts and was quite able to take care of herself if anything happened.

Soon Turner was once again summoning the nursing staff. All the older nurses on the unit turned toward Angie. Angie said: "I'll take care of Mr. Turner. Would anyone like to come with me?" Nobody responded, so Angie walked up to Turner's room, knocked on the door, and asked for permission to enter. Turner was surprised by this approach but not overly impressed. He responded: "Of course, you can come in. How the hell can you get me the remote control from out there?" Angie didn't let it bother her. She entered the room and looked toward the floor at the remote control. She picked it up and handed it to Turner. She asked, "Is there anything else you need Mr. Turner?"

Once again, Turner was surprised by how nice this nurse was acting. At first, he was somewhat disgruntled at the way she was treating him. He wasn't sure if he liked this "nice" nurse. After a couple of nights of taking care of Turner, Angie began to think that the other nurses just weren't treating him properly. Turner began to think that maybe Angie was interested in him. He was actually nice to Angie for a few days, and Angie started to visit him more and more just to make sure he had everything he needed.

One night, after about a week, Turner grabbed Angie and pulled her to the bed. Angie asked what he was doing. Turner replied, "I've been wanting to kiss you for days, and I know you want to kiss me too." With that, Angie jumped up and told Turner that she was a happily married woman and had no intention of kissing him. Turner mumbled something under his breath, but Angie couldn't make out what it was. She left the room. Feeling somewhat embarrassed, Angie decided not to tell anyone what happened. She figured Turner got the message and was not likely to try anything again. Besides, Angie would be off for the next two days.

When Angie returned, everything seemed to be okay for the first couple of days. Turner was not very talkative any more, but Angie figured he was embarrassed by what happened. She was not as nice to him as before either, but she still responded to his call light, gave him his supper and his medications, and accompanied his doc-

tor into the room. Angie decided she would still treat him with dignity and respect, but she wouldn't overdo it by checking on him regularly. She thought that as long as she did her job in a professional manner, everything would be okay.

The next time Angie entered Turner's room, he began to ask her personal questions like: Where do you live? How long have you been married? Are you really happily married? Do you have any kids? Angie was starting to feel a little uneasy about the questions, but she responded with: "I'm sorry, we're not allowed to answer personal questions. It's against our policy." She figured that would make him stop, but it didn't. Each time she entered his room, he became more and more inquisitive, and he began to get angry when Angie wouldn't answer.

One night, Turner overheard two nurses in the corridor talking about how understaffed the unit was that night. That's when he decided he would ring the nurse call button continuously. On the fourth time Angie entered his room that night when Turner said, "I need your help getting on the commode." Since this was pretty routine, Angie never thought much about it, but when she got him into the restroom he locked the door. She reached for the handle, but he grabbed her arm and wouldn't let it go. Turner was a strong man. She thought she could reach the call string next to the commode, but when she tried to grab it, it wasn't there. Turner had removed it earlier in the day.

All of a sudden, Turner grabbed Angie by the throat and started to tug on her clothes. Because Angie was well trained, she immediately put Turner in a wristlock and took him to the floor. Turner cut his lip as he went to the floor and ended up with a sprained wrist. Angie shouted for help. One of the aides heard her shout and went to Turner's room. Angie told her to call security. When security arrived, they took Turner back to his bed. Another nurse came in and treated Turner for his injuries. Before leaving, security complimented Angie on how well she handled the situation.

• • • • • • • • • •

As with any use-of-force situation, Angie had mounds of paperwork to complete. Everyone, including her supervisor, complimented her on how well she handled the situation. She even got a letter of commendation from the hospital CEO.

All's well that ends well, right? Wrong! Could this situation possibly be viewed as controversial? You bet. What happens if/when the patient files a lawsuit? Will the hospital support the nurse's actions? Should they? Since Angie was a well-trained martial artist, couldn't she have done something else that wouldn't have caused injury to the patient? Should the hospital have provided additional training for Angie? And don't forget, there are still those people who believe that a caregiver should never be allowed to use force against a patient, *under any circumstance.*

Introduction

There is a strong correlation between this chapter and Chapter 7. *Like Chapter 7, it is still highly recommended that healthcare providers attend a training course conducted by a competent instructor who specializes in self-defense. In no way should this chapter be construed as a stand-alone training program.* It is important for you to remember that this chapter is based on your right to defend yourself. *The techniques are not to be used in an offensive manner.* You are responsible for knowing the laws in your state as well as your department policy before using any type of force.

All of the basic defensive tactics in the previous chapter still apply. Before beginning the techniques of this chapter, it is important to review some of the basics. First and foremost, understand that the use of these tactics is only to protect the patient, the caregiver, other bystanders, and property. Second, use *only* the minimum amount of force necessary to obtain control of the situation. Third, avoid one-on-one confrontations if at all possible. One-on-one confrontations increase the likelihood of serious injury to the caregiver and the patient.

Throughout this chapter, you will notice that most of the takedowns end with the aggressor lying face down on his or her stomach. This is a critical finale to a takedown for the safety of the caregiver. In the face down position, the aggressor has minimal opportunities to inflict any harm on the caregiver. If the aggressor is left lying face up, he or she can easily hit, bite, kick, scratch, or spit on the caregiver. In the face down position, the aggressor has minimal chances of taking any of these aggressive actions against the caregiver and the caregiver's safety is enhanced. As we will stress throughout this chapter, reasonable caution must be exercised in the use of force by the caregiver and the *reasonable person* standard must always be invoked. Whenever possible, wait for assistance from co-workers, police, security, or other emergency responders.

Whenever you approach any patient, remember to maintain a proper stance. The initial interview stance is accomplished by standing with your feet approximately shoulder width apart, knees slightly bent, and hands held up near chest level. This stance is important for maintaining balance and fending off sudden attacks. If a patient becomes agitated or exhibits any signs of impending violence, switch your feet to the ready stance. This is achieved by moving your strong-side foot back one step, with your foot pointed out at about a 45-degree angle. Your knees remain slightly bent. Your weight should be evenly distributed between both legs, and your head over the center of your body. Your hands should remain up at approximately chest level. Every technique in this chapter is executed from these foundational stances. To help demonstrate the importance of keeping your hands up near chest level and why this stance is so critical, try this little experiment.

Ask a co-worker, friend, relative, or someone else you trust to be your partner. Ask your partner to stand approximately two or three feet away. Place your hands in your pockets. Ask your partner to throw a punch toward your face. *It is not necessary to actually receive the punch.* See how long it takes you to get your hands out of your pocket to block the punch. Chances are, you won't be able to get your hands out of your pockets before the punch is delivered. Now try it with your hands up at chest level. Typically, reaction time is greatly improved in this position.

Next, have your partner stand directly in front of you. Place your feet together. Ask your partner to push you backward, using the least amount of pressure needed to accomplish the task. With your feet together, it should not take much pressure to move you. Place your feet together again. Ask your partner to stand at your side and again exert only the least amount of force necessary to move you off balance sideways. Once again, the amount of pressure necessary was probably minimal. Now, get into your ready stance. Bend your knees slightly more than in the interview stance, and ask your partner to attempt to push you again. This time your partner needs to exert much more force to push you, if you can be moved at all.

The duration of this chapter is designed to provide healthcare providers with the basic knowledge needed to block several types of kicks and punches. In addition, information on escort holds and controlled takedowns will be shared. There is no way to show every type of kick, grab, or punch you may encounter. Every situation is unique. One of the best ways to learn these techniques is to teach them to others. The more you learn, teach, and practice the techniques presented, the more likely you will be to retain them for future use.

Blocking Kicks

Kicks, grabs, and punches are often sudden and unexpected. But whether they are sudden and unexpected, or slowly telegraphed, the best way to block any type of kick, grab, or punch is to always anticipate the possibility of violence. The importance of advance preparation and planning can't be stressed enough. If you plan for, anticipate, and practice what you will do before a violent episode occurs, your reaction time will be improved, you will have more confidence, and the possibility of serious injury will be minimized. If you can't find someone to practice with, practice by yourself. As you go about your normal day, conducting business as usual, play out several scenarios in your mind. For example, as you are completing your paperwork, think about what you would do if a violent person suddenly confronted you. If you react properly during your scenario, odds are you will act properly if the real situation occurs. This works with all types of situations. As you are en route to the scene of an accident, think through how you would handle the situation if the patient refused treatment and became belligerent. The more types of situations you come up with, the better prepared you'll be to handle them. The same thing works with kicks, grabs, and punches.

There are several types of kicks, and we will try to cover as many as possible; however, it is important to realize that these techniques may have to be modified according to the situation. Every violent encounter is unique. It is also important to note that an attack does not normally end when the initial kick, grab, or punch is blocked. In each of these situations, remember to keep your head protected at all times and remain ready for the next attack. No matter what type of kick an aggressor uses, it will end up in one of three places—low, middle, or high on your body. With this in mind, there are three basic kick blocks from two different stances—the low kick block, middle kick block, and high kick block from the interview stance and from the defensive stance. These blocks may be used on the right side of the body, the left side of the body, or directly in front of the body.

Low Kick Block from the Interview Stance

When you are in the interview stance, most likely you are not anticipating an aggressive action. One of the best ways to defend against a low kick is to immediately react by stepping back with the leg directly opposite of the aggressor's kicking leg, which will force the aggressor off balance. While keeping your weight on that leg, raise the opposite side knee toward the center of your body, so your leg is bent at about a 90-degree angle, and block the kick with the outside part of the weak leg.

Middle Kick Block from the Interview Stance

For an aggressor to kick toward the middle portion of your body, he or she has to point their knee to the area of the body they plan to kick. Once again, take a step back with the leg directly opposite the aggressor's kicking leg. Bring the opposite leg up toward the center of your body. At the same time, cross both arms over your chest, tuck your elbows in tightly to protect the upper portion of your middle body, and block the kick with your arms.

High Kick Block from the Interview Stance

Once again, an aggressor will have to point his or her knee toward the intended target. As soon as you see the knee start to rise, take a step back with the leg directly opposite the aggressor's kicking leg. Turn your body toward the raised knee. While maintaining your balance, tuck your chin down toward your chest as much as possible, and raise your arms together to protect your head and upper body. It is important that you continue to keep your eyes on the aggressor and after the kick is blocked continue to back up, putting yourself in a better defensive position.

Low Kick Block from the Defensive Stance

In a proper defensive stance, simply pivot your leg inward on the side from which the aggressor is kicking. At the same time, shift all of your body weight to the opposite leg. Then bring one arm down and over the groin to protect the middle part of your body. Keep your other arm up to protect your head in case the aggressor follows through with another kick or a punch. For example, if the aggressor is kicking with his or her right leg, pivot your left leg toward the middle of your body, put all of your weight on your right leg, lower your left arm to protect your groin, and keep your right arm up near your face to protect your head. Always assume that an aggressor will continue the attack, regardless of whether you blocked the initial kick or not.

Middle Kick Block from the Defensive Stance

For an aggressor to kick toward the middle portion of your body, he or she has to point their knee to the area of the body they plan to kick. Once again, take a step back with the leg directly opposite the aggressor's kicking leg. Bring your opposite leg up toward the center of your body. At the same time, cross both your arms over your chest, tuck your elbows in tightly to protect the upper portion of your middle body, and block the kick with your arms.

High Kick Block from the Defensive Stance

Once again, an aggressor will have to point his or her knee toward the intended target to accomplish this kick. As soon as you see the aggressor's knee start to rise, take a step back with the leg directly opposite the aggressor's leg. Turn your body toward the raised knee. While maintaining your balance, tuck your chin down toward your chest as much as possible, and raise your arms together to protect your head and upper body. It is important that you continue to keep your eyes on the aggressor and after the kick is blocked, continue to back up, putting yourself in a better defensive position.

Blocking Punches

Punches are much the same as grabs, except that they are normally delivered quicker and with more force, making them more difficult to defend against. Once again, maintaining the correct stance and distance, and keeping your hands up near chest level, will increase the odds that you can effectively defend against a punch. For the purpose of this chapter, the focus will be on the best defense against the type of punch being thrown rather than protecting the area of the body targeted.

Roundhouse Punch

A roundhouse punch may be blocked to the inside or the outside, depending on the situation. The best way to defend against a roundhouse punch is to take a step back and to the same side from which the punch is being delivered, basically staying outside the reach of the aggressor. Lean your body away from the punch while raising the hand opposite the direction of the lean. Redirect the aggressor's punch away from your body, bringing the aggressor off balance. You should end up almost directly behind the aggressor after your follow-through. If you find there is not enough time or room to get outside of the aggressor's reach, raise your arm at about a 45-degree angle on the side from which the aggressor is delivering the punch. Next, step in toward the aggressor and block the punch with the outside part of your arm. Stepping in toward the aggressor will minimize the leverage of the punch, and the punch will be absorbed by your arm and body.

Straight Punch

A straight punch is extremely difficult to defend against. If an aggressor is punching straight at you, take a step back, keep your hands open, and slap the aggressor's elbow toward the inside of their body.

Backfist Punch

A backfist punch is normally delivered to the side or to the top of the body. If it is delivered to the side, bring both your arms up at a 90-degree angle, elbows chest high with your forearms and hands protecting your face and head (see Figure 8-1). If it is delivered to the top, bring both arms up to protect your head and block the punch with your elbows and forearms (see Figure 8-2).

Escorting Uncooperative Patients

From time to time the healthcare provider may be called upon to escort an individual to a location he or she doesn't want to go. Sometimes the individual is compliant; other times the individual, although not violent, is passive aggressive. They aren't fully uncooperative, they are simply being defensive to the caregiver's effort to help. When this occurs, you need to verbally communicate to the individual that you are there to help and that you need their cooperation. If the individual does not respond to you, you are now faced with several decisions to make. Should you contact the police for assistance? Should you call for additional support from other caregivers? Do you have the right, or the responsibility, to treat the patient

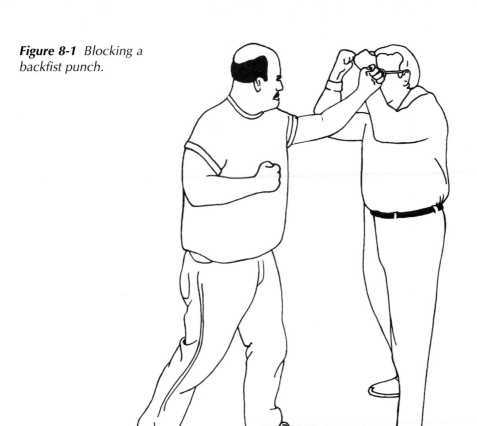

Figure 8-1 *Blocking a backfist punch.*

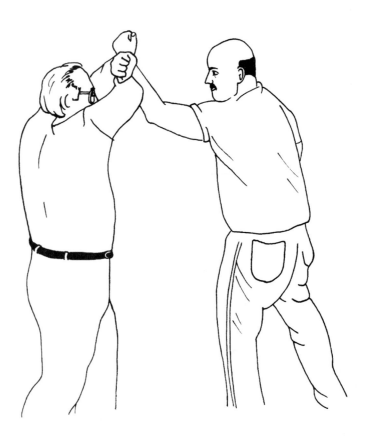

Figure 8-2 *Blocking a backfist punch delivered to the top.*

against his or her will? Does the patient have the right to refuse treatment? If so, has the patient actually refused? These are questions that should be answered before you make any decision. Assume for the time being that you decide to escort the patient to the desired location. You grab the patient and begin escorting him or her to the location. By turning a defensive situation into an offensive one, have you just committed battery against the patient? There is no easy way to answer some of these questions. However, the best answer is to know the laws in your jurisdiction and your company policy and to apply them along with the reasonable person standard, in consideration of the total circumstances of the situation. Where it may be reasonable to escort a minor against his or her will, with the parent's permission, it may not be reasonable to escort a fully competent adult against his or her will. In many cases, the physician and/or local law enforcement may be called upon to make this decision.

Once the decision to escort an individual has been made, you need to do it in a safe manner, meaning a manner that is safe for the patient as well as for yourself. One way to escort someone to a desired location is to place your hand over his or her wrist. Always use your hand on the same side as theirs. For example, if you are controlling their left wrist, use your left hand. Take your opposite hand and place it directly above their elbow, palm side in and thumb up. Apply a minimal amount of pressure above their elbow to elicit the cooperation needed. If the patient becomes combative, simply step toward them, pushing him or her away from you, while preparing yourself for a possible attack. This escort works extremely well when done as a team. With one person on the left side and one person on the right side of the patient, he or she can be easily directed to the desired location with minimal force.

Takedowns

On occasion, you may encounter a patient who, for whatever reason, continues grabbing and punching at you regardless of your efforts to bring calm to the situation or de-escalate the hostility. The only way to keep the patient from hurting himself, yourself, bystanders, or property, is to take the patient to the ground and physically restrain them. In an ideal world, the best way to accomplish this is to contact the local police for assistance. However, since this is the real world, there may be a number of reasons why you can't wait for the police to arrive. The police may be several minutes away and waiting for them may serve to aggravate the situation even further. The individual may have grabbed you, another caregiver, or a bystander, forcing you to react to protect them. The individual may be attempting to hurt him- or herself, elevating the severity of the situation and causing you to provide a more immediate response. Whatever the reason, should you have to take an individual to the ground from either a grab or a punch, you will again want to do it in the safest manner possible. Every takedown in this text is a "controlled takedown," meaning that you will do everything in your power to protect yourself, others around you, and the patient you are controlling to the ground.

Takedown from a One-Hand Wrist Grab

When someone grabs you by the wrist, a common immediate reaction is to pull away, which often causes more injury. Instead, when someone grabs you by the wrist, step back slightly to bring him or her off balance. As soon as they are off balance, distract them by pinching, slapping toward their eyes with your free hand, or by shouting in a distinct tone. Next, open your hand that is being grabbed by the aggressor and turn it upward and around the outside of the aggressor's wrist. (By opening your hand you have strengthened your wrist and made it harder for the aggressor to maintain his or her grip.) Grab the aggressor's arm with your other hand directly above their wrist to trap them. Tuck your elbows in tightly toward your stomach and bend forward, exerting only the minimal amount of pressure to bring the aggressor to the ground. Do not let go of the aggressor's arm; without applying additional pressure, maintain control of their wrist. Give loud, repetitive commands to the aggressor so he or she will know what you want them to do. Ask the aggressor to lay on their stomach. Do not become complacent. Keep control. If the aggressor begins to struggle, apply enough pressure to elicit their cooperation. Call for assistance.

Takedown from a Two-Hand Wrist Grab

If you happen to get grabbed by both wrists, the same maneuver applied in the one-hand wrist grab may be used. Again, step back slightly to bring the aggressor off balance. As soon as they are off balance, open either of your hands that are being grabbed by the aggressor, and turn it upward and around to grab the outside of the aggressor's wrist. Distract them by shouting very loudly in a distinct tone. When they are distracted, break your other hand free and place it on the aggressor's arm directly in front of the hand on the aggressor's wrist. Tuck your elbows in tightly toward your stomach and bend forward, exerting only the minimal amount of pressure to bring the aggressor to the ground. Do not let go of the aggressor's arm; without applying additional pressure, maintain control of their wrist. Give loud, repetitive commands to the aggressor so that he or she will know what you want him or her to do. Ask the aggressor to lay on their stomach. Do not become complacent. Keep control. If the aggressor begins to struggle, apply enough pressure to elicit their cooperation. Call for assistance.

Takedown from a Front Hair Grab

The normal reaction to being grabbed by the hair is to jerk away. Jerking away can cause severe pain and discomfort, not to mention hair loss. If someone places you in a front hair grab, immediately put both of your hands over the aggressor's hand to trap it tightly to your head. This maneuver will keep the aggressor from being able to pull your hair out. Next, take a step back to take the aggressor off balance, then turn your body, placing your elbow against the aggressor's elbow and continue turning into the elbow and downward until the aggressor is on the ground (refer to Figures 7-7a and 7-7b). Do not let go of the aggressor's arm; without applying additional pressure, maintain control of their wrist. Ask the aggressor to lay on their stomach. Do not become complacent. Keep control. If the aggressor begins to struggle, apply enough pressure to elicit their cooperation. Call for assistance.

Takedown from a Rear Hair Grab

If someone grabs your hair from the rear, avoid the reaction to pull away. Place both of your hands over the aggressor's hand to trap it tightly to your head. Next, take a step forward to take the aggressor off balance, then turn your body into the aggressor's elbow and continue turning into the elbow and downward until the aggressor loses their grip (refer to Figures 7-8a and 7-8b). With your forearm nearest the aggressor's body, apply downward pressure just above the elbow, while maintaining control of their wrist with your other hand. Once the aggressor is on the ground ask them to lie on their stomach. Do not let go; maintain control of their wrist without applying additional pressure. Do not become complacent. Keep control. If the aggressor begins to struggle, apply enough pressure to elicit their cooperation. Call for assistance.

Takedown from a Clothing Grab

Many times an aggressor will grab your shirt at the lapel in an attempt to intimidate you. Once again, resist the urge to pull away. Instead, place one hand over the aggressor's, locking it in place. Take your free hand and distract the aggressor by pinching the underside of their arm, slapping toward their eyes, or by shouting in a distinct tone. Simultaneously, peel the offender's hand away from your shirt, turning their wrist in an inward or outward motion. Use your free hand to lock the aggressor's arm at the elbow until you get the aggressor to the ground (refer to Figures 7-9a, 7-9b, and 7-9c). Ask the aggressor to lay on their stomach. Do not let go; maintain control of their wrist without applying additional pressure. Do not become complacent. Keep control. If the aggressor begins to struggle, apply enough pressure to elicit their cooperation. Call for assistance.

Another common clothing grab involves the aggressor putting their hand against your chest, palm in, and grabbing at your shirt. Immediately place both of your hands over the aggressor's hand to trap it in place, then bend at the waist toward the aggressor and downward until the aggressor goes down to the ground. Once the aggressor is on the ground, ask them to lie on their stomach. Do not let go; maintain control of their wrist without applying additional pressure. Do not become complacent. Keep control. If the aggressor begins to struggle, apply enough pressure to elicit their cooperation. Call for assistance.

Takedown from a Roundhouse Punch

As the aggressor punches toward you, raise your arm at about a 45-degree angle on the same side from which the aggressor is delivering the punch, step in toward the aggressor, and block the punch with the outside part of your arm. Redirect the punch to continue through until it is against your side. With the arm you used to block the punch, wrap your arm around the aggressor's arm and exert upward pressure against their elbow. With your foot farthest from the aggressor (remember, you are in a defensive stance), step behind the aggressor's foot on the same side as the arm you have wrapped. (If you have his right arm wrapped, step your right leg behind his right leg.) With your free hand, apply pressure to the brachial plexus tie-in, which is located where the shoulder meets the body, pushing backward until the aggressor is lowered to the ground. With your arm wrapped around the aggressor's arm, you should be able to control the takedown such that the aggressor does not hit their head. When the aggressor is on the ground on their back, take your free hand again and apply pressure just below the aggressor's elbow, turning them on their stomach. Do not let go; maintain control of their wrist without applying additional pressure. Do not become complacent. Keep control. If the aggressor begins to struggle, apply enough pressure to elicit their cooperation. Call for assistance.

Takedown from a Straight Punch

If an aggressor is punching straight at you, take a step back, keeping your hands open. With your hand on the inside of the aggressor's punch, redirect the punch away from you, while grabbing on to their wrist. Let the aggressor continue the follow through and when he or she stops, take your free hand and place it over your other hand, bringing the aggressor's wrist back upward. Continue to turn the aggressor's wrist inward until he or she is controlled to the ground. Do not let go of the aggressor's wrist. When the aggressor is on the ground on their back, again take your free hand and apply pressure just below the aggressor's elbow, turning them on their stomach. Maintain control of their wrist without applying additional pressure. Do not become complacent. Keep control. If the aggressor begins to struggle, apply enough pressure to elicit their cooperation. Call for assistance.

Summary

Once again, remember that these techniques are not all inclusive. The number and types of blocks, grabs, and punches are only limited by the mind. Every person has their own unique style of fighting, whether they are highly skilled martial artists or common street fighters. Learn these defensive techniques, practice them as often as possible, and modify them to fit each situation appropriately.

Types and Uses
of Restraints

Just Another Drunk . . .

It was as simple a dispatch as any of the hundreds he had been on . . . an ambulance requested by the police at a local tavern for an "uncooperative subject."

With 15 years of experience as a paramedic, Tony Milano had responded to calls like this too many times to get excited. He could almost describe the scene before the ambulance ever left the firehouse . . . "police called to a local establishment for a patron getting loud and obscene . . . police arrive at the scene, nobody wants to sign a complaint, they just want the individual removed . . . individual is too intoxicated to drive . . . has no ID . . . police can't take him to jail, as he has had too much to drink . . . so call an ambulance and take him to the local ER to dry out . . ."

Upon arrival at the scene, Tony saw exactly what he expected. Two police cars in the parking lot, with the "patient" leaning against one of them in an attempt to stay upright. What surprised Tony was that this was not the "patient" he had expected. This patient was female, in her mid-forties, moderately built, and obviously fond of the bottle. As he approached the patient, Tony heard her utter "whatch a ambulash fer?" Laughter from the police was the only response she received.

"Rose, these guys are going to take you to the hospital so you can sober up, and then you will be able to come back, get your car, and go home."

"Hoshpidal—I ain't goin to no damn hoshpidal," she argued, "I ain't shick."

"But Rose, you know the routine. Go to the ER, sleep it off, and go home in the morning."

"Really—thatsh all?"

"Yes Rose, that's all. Why don't you jump up here on the stretcher, and let these guys check you out, then they will take you in."

"Shure, zish one's kinda cute anyway," she said, grabbing onto Tony's arm. "I'd go anywhere wish hims."

With Tony's help, Rose willingly climbed onto the stretcher and was placed in the back of the ambulance. When Tony placed the safety belt around her waist, she started to resist, but quickly quieted down when he agreed to only use one safety belt instead of three and would leave her arms and upper body unrestrained.

En route to the hospital, a 15-minute ride, Tony attempted to make small talk with Rose. For some reason, she did not seem to be the "happy drunk" she had been while the police were present. Now she kept mumbling about "don't need no damn doctors or no rotten hoshpidal." At one point, she looked at Tony and stated, "Ya know hot shot, I's could get outa here in no time if I wanted to, and you couldn't do shkwuat to schtop me."

Trying not to laugh, Tony replied, "I know, Rose . . ."

A few miles down the road, circumstances changed. "I ain't going to no damn hoshpidal—I'm getting out here now." With that, she began attempting to undo the safety belt on the stretcher.

"Hold it Rose . . ." Tony started, as he leaned over her to grab her wrist—then suddenly everything changed. As he leaned across her, the patient leaned forward and bit him on the ear, in effect biting off a piece of his lower lobe. Tony heard himself scream and felt the blood run down his neck. As he grabbed at his ear, the patient reached out and scratched his face, barely missing his eyes. As his partner pulled the ambulance over, Tony bailed out the side door, holding his ear and face. At the same time, the intoxicated patient finished freeing herself from the one restraint and was able to open the back door of the ambulance, and escape into the darkness. With the assistance of his partner, Tony was stabilized and transported to the ER for treatment. The police later arrested the intoxicated patient at her home.

• • • • • • • • • •

Episodes like this one are not uncommon. Prehospital providers, understandably hoping to avoid confrontation with an intoxicated or belligerent patient, bend the rules in an attempt to keep the patient calm. Unfortunately, their efforts, no matter how noble in intent, come back to haunt them.

In our scenario, several mistakes were made by the provider, which led to his injury. How many did you recognize? Perhaps they included the following:

1. Allowing the patient to "snuggle up" to him at the scene
2. Only placing one safety belt on the patient, despite having three on the cot
3. Leaning across in front of the patient's face in an attempt to stop her from releasing the single safety belt

The professional healthcare worker, whether in the prehospital, acute care, or long-term care setting, must always be prepared to deal with the unexpected and must realize that every patient has the potential to cause harm to him or her.

Introduction

There are as many types of restraint devices on the healthcare market as there are reasons to use them. The use of restraints remains a debated issue. Some feel that, when appropriately used, restraints offer maximum safety to patients who may otherwise be at risk to fall or to injure themselves or others. Others contend that the use of restraints is inhumane and is a violation of the patient's rights. Whether you have a bias on the use of restraint devices or not, it is incumbent upon you to know the ways in which they are intended to be used. They must also be used according to local, state, and federal laws and in a way that maximizes safety for the patient and staff.

Throughout this chapter, when we use the term *restraint* we will use the following definition: *any method of physically restricting a person's freedom of movement, physical activity, or access to his or her body.*

Purpose of Restraints

Before talking about the actual purpose and use of restraint devices, it is important to note that restraints are not to be used to punish patients nor for staff convenience. Let's repeat that: restraints are not to be used to punish patients nor for staff convenience. Providing quality healthcare, whether it is in the prehospital, the acute care, or the long-term care setting, is based on meeting the needs of the patient. Nowhere is "punishment" defined as a form of medical treatment (apart from certain behavioral environments). When restraints are used as a way to control an aggressive patient, the healthcare provider must always remember that the patient is only being restrained to protect him- or herself from injury and not for punishment based on the behaviors exhibited.

Whenever it is necessary to restrain a patient, it is incumbent upon the healthcare professional to clearly document the reasoning behind the use of restraints, including the behaviors demonstrated by the patient before the decision to use a restraint device. The decision to use restraint devices, as well as the documentation following their use, should be evaluated as a part of every departmental organization's ongoing quality improvement process.

Legal Considerations

In almost every arena of healthcare, legislation exists on the use of various types of restraint devices. In the prehospital setting, the use of restraint devices as a method of behavioral control has only been weakly addressed, compared with other areas of healthcare. To the prehospital provider, this is essential. In most cases, when restraints are used in the prehospital setting it is because the patient is out of control, presents a risk of injury to him- or herself, and/or presents a risk of injury to the prehospital provider. Combine these reasons with the tight quarters afforded prehospital providers in the back of an ambulance and the amount of movement and rocking that goes on while it is in motion, and one can appreciate why the use of restraints in the prehospital setting is often significantly higher than in any other form of healthcare.

The hospital environment, on the other hand, is much more regulated in the use of restraint devices. Specific criteria are set forth that staff must consider before applying a restraint device. Unlike an ambulance, where space is limited and staffing is at the bare minimum (often a one-to-one ratio) with no additional help available, hospitals are perceived to have adequate staffing and a greater ability to deal with the aggressive behaviors of patients. Furthermore, hospitals must meet more stringent regulatory standards when considering the use of restraint devices. In hospitals, the Patient Bill of Rights, either explicitly or implicitly gives the patient the right to be free from unreasonable or inhumane restraint. As a result, our hospitals are now forced to spend more time training their people in techniques of aggression management than ever before. Stringent clinical indicators must be met before a patient can be considered a candidate for physical restraint, and even then the restraint device must be the method that is the "least restrictive while most effective."

In nursing homes (and in hospital-affiliated skilled nursing facilities) the use of restraints is very closely monitored and controlled by regulatory agencies. Again, with no disrespect to either school of thought, the use of restraints in caring for and controlling the behavior of the elderly residents is a hotly debated topic. Of all forms of healthcare, long-term care is the area in which the use of restraint devices receives the greatest amount of attention and regulatory agency involvement. In fact, the use of restraints in long-term care facilities is nearly prohibited. The position held by government regulatory agencies is that because a person ages and goes through continuous behavioral changes, the obligation is on the healthcare provider to adapt the environment to meet the changing condition of the resident without restricting the ability of the resident to move or to roam. Federal agencies such as the Health Care Finance Administration have issued regulatory standards on the use of restraints. These standards are very specific on how and when restraints can be used. Failure to comply with these standards could result in loss of Medicare provider status.

Because there are so many legal considerations surrounding the use of restraint devices, the organizations—prehospital, acute care, or long-term care—must research the issue and obtain a legal opinion on the use of restraint devices. This includes identifying the appropriate and acceptable type of restraint devices and ensuring that all staff members are trained in all areas of restraint use and application.

Types of Restraints

Typically restraints are categorized into one of two categories: chemical restraints and physical restraints.

Chemical Restraints

Chemical restraints are medications that are given to a patient through intravenous or intramuscular injection, by oral administration, or by absorption through the skin. Chemical restraints are designed in such a way that, when administered in the appropriate dose, they alter the patient's behavior to the point in which they are no longer a threat to themselves or others around them. Often these chemicals work by inducing sleep, by sedation, or by depressing the central nervous system.

Chemical restraints require an order from a physician before administration. Some of the more common drugs used as chemical restraints include Ativan, Haldol, Librium, Thorazine, and Valium.

In modern healthcare, the swing of the pendulum has now gone away from the use of chemical restraints, at least from the degree that they once were used. When chemical restraints are used, clinicians are urged to use weaker dosages than they did in the past, and certainly with lesser frequency. With the development of newer and better drugs, the use of chemical therapy as a restraint tool has decreased; instead, prescription medications, taken on a regular basis, help to control behaviors of the aggressive patient in such a way that chemical restraint in a crisis has become less common and less necessary.

Physical Restraints

Much as the name implies, physical restraints are devices that are designed to be physically applied to the patient with the intent of limiting their mobility. Traditionally, physical restraint devices have fallen into one of five categories:

- Jacket restraint (vest restraint)
- Belt restraint
- Extremity restraint
- Mitten restraint
- Elbow restraint

Each type of physical restraint device has an intended use, and it is up to the healthcare provider to know each device, understand its intended use, and be able to demonstrate proficiency in its proper use and application. Let's look at each device in greater detail.

Jacket Restraint (Vest Restraint)

The jacket or vest restraint has traditionally been used in attempts to manage patients who have been commonly referred to as "wanderers." Wanderers are patients who have a tendency to get up and wander to various locations throughout the facility and even onto the grounds. Jacket or vest restraints are uncommon in the prehospital setting because the total immobility of the device causes injuries to patients who try to free themselves from it. For years they were very common in both hospitals and nursing homes to prevent patients from wandering out of the building and into harms way.

Today, the jacket restraint is rarely used. Many patients have been injured because jacket restraints were incorrectly applied by healthcare providers. If this device is not properly applied, serious orthopedic injury may result to the patient. If the patient has dementia, or any other type of degenerative or organic brain disease, the risk of injury from this device becomes even greater, as the patient is unable to appreciate the injury that they may cause themselves by trying to escape from the device.

Another hazard of this device is that often the patient is able to reach the straps that are used to secure the device in place. Patients have been seriously injured because they were able to reach the straps, untie them, escape from the device, and subsequently fall and injure themselves.

Jacket restraints, although once quite popular, should be used with caution and hesitation. A safer form of patient management should be considered.

Belt Restraint

In hospitals and nursing homes alike, the use of belt restraints was once as common place as an IV pole. Belt restraints were preferred by many healthcare providers because of the ease with which they worked, and because they could be used in a bed and in a wheelchair or a straight chair. The belt restraint was simply a device that attached to the frame of the bed or the chair and went across the patient's waist, securing them to the bed or the chair. Unfortunately, the belt restraint, when used by itself, created what some argue was a greater hazard than the use of no restraint device at all (see Figure 9-1).

One of the greatest hazards of the belt restraint was the risk of suffocation or strangulation to the patient. When simply used as a belt across the waist in a hospital bed, most patients became very agitated by the presence of the belt. Many patients, especially those small and frail in stature, were able to easily maneuver themselves out from under the belt restraint device and "escape" to freedom. Unfortunately, many of these patients sustained injuries in the process.

Even worse, there are documented cases in which patients attempted to crawl out from under the belt restraint device and tragically ended up with the restraint device around their neck, essentially hanging themselves on the belt.

The same hazards exist when using a belt restraint device in a wheelchair or a straight chair. When the belt is applied around the patient's waist in a chair, the natural tendency of the patient when trying to escape

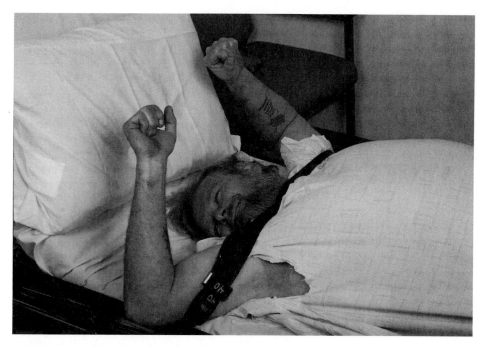

Figure 9-1 *Patients have been injured and killed by belt restraints. These restraints must be used cautiously.*

is to try to slide out of the chair under the belt. Again, this has caused many tragic deaths.

When evaluating the appropriate type of restraint device to be used on a patient, the belt restraint device, like the jacket or vest restraint, must be used very cautiously and only when more appropriate forms of restraint devices are not available.

Extremity Restraint

Much as the name implies, extremity restraint devices are those devices that are designed to reduce or eliminate the patient's ability to use their extremities. Extremity restraint devices are among the most effective physical restraint devices on the market today. Because of the way in which they work, they are also one of the most debated and contested forms of physical restraint devices.

One of the nicest features of the extremity restraint device is its ability to control how many extremities are immobilized and how immobile the extremities are rendered. Depending on the amount of aggression demonstrated by the patient, and the amount of physical restraint required, extremity restraint devices can be applied on one, two, three, or all four extremities. They work well in both the prehospital and the acute-care setting, but the use of extremity restraint devices is frowned upon in long-term care settings.

Caution must be exercised when choosing the restraint device. Using the wrong type may result in avoidable injury to the patient or to the healthcare provider (see Figure 9-2). For example, if the patient is combative and extremity restraints are necessary, "soft" restraints, such as those used to prevent falls, would not be appropriate. The patient can easily break free from these and cause injury to him- or herself or others. On the other hand, if the restraint device is needed to limit mobility or prevent a fall, then leather restraints would be inappropriate.

Types of Restraints

Mitten Restraint

Mittens are a form of restraint device used to control a patient's behavior without limiting his or her mobility. Mittens, just as the name implies, are used over the hands of the patient when they have a tendency to scratch or grab at providers or when they may be inclined to inflict pain upon themselves by repeated scratching, gouging, or other similar forms of self-abuse. Beyond these uses mitten restraints do not provide an effective form of control.

Elbow Restraint

Seldom used in modern healthcare, elbow restraints were once commonly used as a behavioral control technique. These devices, when properly applied, "locked" the arm in a straight position and prevented the patient from bending the elbow. The arms could then be secured to the frame of

Figure 9-2 Extremity restraint devices should be selected based on the reason they are being used. Use of the wrong type greatly increases the risk of injury to the patient and the provider.

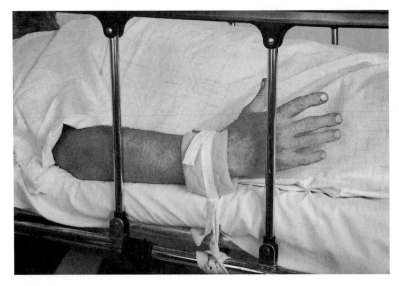

Soft restraint

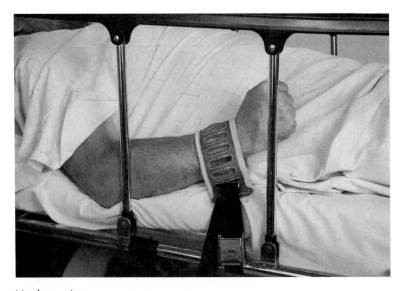

Hard restraint

Chapter 9: Types and Uses of Restraints

the patient's bed. This form of restraint is often seen as excessive and there are now better techniques on the market that have resulted in near extinction of elbow restraint devices.

Application and Use of Restraints

In applying restraints on a patient, we use the term *point* to describe the number of locations at which the patient is restrained. Typically, restraint devices are applied using anywhere from a one-point to a six-point technique, depending upon the type of restraint device being used and reason for it. Some of these techniques are intended for very short-term use while others are intended to completely immobilize the patient until he or she is able to regain control of him- or herself.

One-Point Restraint

A one-point restraint is a temporary restraint technique. It is not meant to exercise physical control of an aggressive patient, nor is it intended as a restraint technique in order to leave a patient unattended for any reason. More often than not, the most common reason for its use is a therapeutic one, such as accessing an IV sight. Once the task is accomplished, the one-point restraint is released (see Figure 9-3).

The application of a one-point restraint for purposes of patient control is inappropriate. The use of a one-point restraint for gaining patient control will result in one of two things: (1) either the patient will release themselves from the restraint, or (2) the patient will sustain serious orthopedic injury in his or her attempt to remove the restraint.

Two-Point Restraint

Two-point restraint refers to a technique by which either both arms, both legs, or one of each on the same side or alternate sides is restrained. Much like the one-point restraint, the two-point restraint presents serious risk to the patient and to the provider if used inappropriately. The two-point technique can be used to restrain:

- Both arms
- Both legs
- One arm and one leg

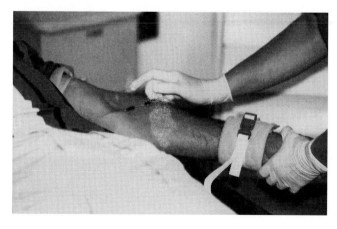

Figure 9-3 The one-point restraint device can be used to support therapeutic care but should not be used for patient control purposes.

When both arms are restrained, a patient's upper body may be immobilized but both legs remain free and can easily be used to kick at the provider. When both legs are restrained, the patient may be unable to flee from the bed or the stretcher but since both hands are left free, the patient can grab, strike, push, or hold the provider. In addition, drunken or delusional patients in two-point leg restraints have been known to get up off of the bed and have thereby fallen to the floor, sustaining serious injury (see Figure 9-4).

Some individuals prefer to use a two-point restraint to immobilize alternating upper and lower extremities, for instance right arm/left leg or left arm/right leg. Although this immobilizes the upper and lower torso, it still presents risk of injury to both the patient and the provider because one arm and one leg are free at all times.

Three-Point Restraint

The three-point restraint is another physical restraint technique that can be adapted a number of ways to accomplish the following:

- Immobilization using two arm restraints and one leg restraint
- Immobilization using two leg restraints and one arm restraint
- Immobilization using one arm restraint, one leg restraint, and one middle body restraint, such as a belt restraint device
- Immobilization using a chest restraint (belt), a waist restraint (belt), and a leg restraint

Many of the same hazards addressed in the discussion of the two-point restraint are again present in the three-point restraint. The three-point restraint is not recommended for use in behavioral control except in those rare cases in which no other form is available or if it will only be used temporarily until a better method becomes available.

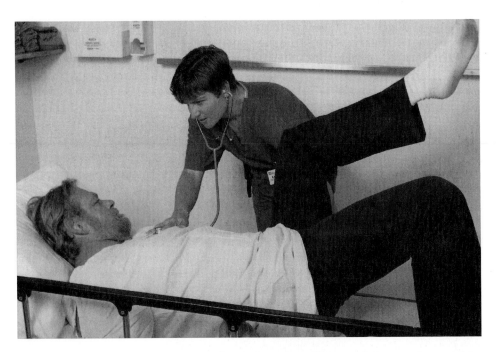

Figure 9-4 *In a two-point restraint, the patient can still cause injury to the provider using his arm or leg.*

Chapter 9: Types and Uses of Restraints

Four-Point Restraint

The four-point restraint is probably the most common restraint technique. In the four-point restraint, both upper and lower extremities are immobilized. Although immobilizing all four extremities may give the provider the sense of safety and well-being, it must be recognized that there are many hazards associated with this technique, presenting risk to both the patient and the provider (see Figure 9-5).

Positioning is the most vital issue when talking about the four-point restraint. When using this technique, the legs will normally be placed in one of two positions, either side by side or crossed. Side by side is obviously the more humane of the two and presents the least risk of injury to the patient. The use of the cross-leg technique should be avoided whenever possible. If it is necessary, it is appropriate that a physician evaluate the patient to ensure that the patient's positioning will not compromise or exacerbate his or her medical conditions or treatment.

There are a number of positions that the upper extremities can be placed in when using a four-point restraint. The most common is to place the patient's arms at their side with the restraint device secured to the bed frame. This position provides the greatest mobility to the patient while restrained, because the patient is still able to sit up and move their upper torso freely above the bed or the stretcher. That is not to say that this position does not present risk to both the patient and the provider. When in this position, the patient, if able to sit up, can use his or her skull to strike at the provider. Even worse, the patient may be able to inflict serious biting injuries to the provider.

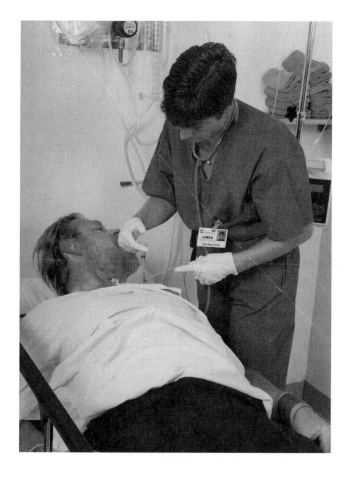

Figure 9-5 Even in a four-point restraint, the patient may be able to bite the provider or use his head to strike out at the provider.

Another technique is to place both the patient's hands above their head while they are laying on the bed, with the restraint device then applied to the head of the bed. In this position, the patient's arms are extended above their head. *We highly discourage this technique* because the patient may sustain serious orthopedic injury if he or she begins to rise up off of the bed. When resistance is met, the patient may tug harder and harder, ultimately causing serious injury to their shoulders, arms, back, chest, or neck.

Yet another technique, which was once commonly taught, is a modified side arm position by which both upper extremities are left down at the patient's side and then crossed over the abdomen. This position lessens the ability of the patient to sit up in bed and to use his or her head or mouth as a weapon against the provider. Because the patient's arms are crossed diagonally over the chest and abdomen, access to the chest and abdomen for medical treatment or radiological procedures may be limited if not prohibited. Thus, it is obvious why this technique is seldom used and why more preferred techniques are sought out.

Still another technique to restrain the upper extremities is the hi-low technique. In this technique, one arm is elevated and secured above the head, while the other arm is secured at the patient's side. As a result, the patient is immobilized and unable to use the upper body as a weapon, and one of the two lower extremities remains accessible for medical treatment purposes such as IV access. It is important that the healthcare provider, whether in the prehospital or hospital setting, remember that in this position, the patient should be continuously monitored and his or her extremities rotated at least every 15 minutes. If this is not done, injury may result to the patient.

Five-Point Restraint

The use of the five-point restraint is another technique that is used only under extreme circumstances and only for short periods of time.

The five-point restraint technique involves the use of traditional four-point restraints as previously discussed, with the addition of a chest strap placed across the patient's chest and under his or her arms to further immobilize the patient and restrict body movement. Again, it must be emphasized that this technique should only be used in extreme circumstances and only for short periods of time.

Six-Point Restraint

The sixth and final technique, the six-point restraint, involves all the techniques introduced in the five-point restraint, with the addition of a sixth point in the form of a restraint belt across the patient's legs above the knees. Again, this technique should only be used in the most extreme circumstances and is intended for short-term use only (see Figure 9-6).

Special Considerations

Any time a special restraint device is used to control a patient certain considerations must be made. Some of these considerations are made well in advance, while others must be made at the time that the provider is dealing with the patient. Discussions of these special considerations follow.

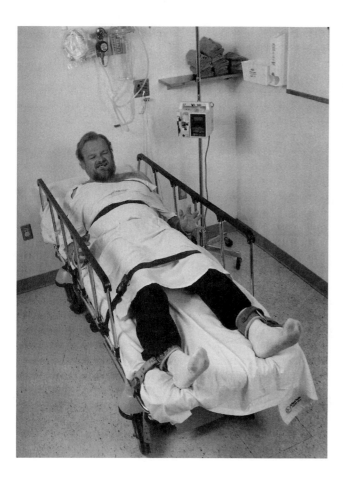

Figure 9-6 *Six-point restraint offers maximum control and should only be used when all else fails.*

Positioning

Extreme caution must always be taken when considering positions for restraining an aggressive patient. Patients should always be restrained on their backs. Under no circumstances should a patient be restrained face down. This is often a point of debate and concern when both police agencies and prehospital agencies are interacting with the same patient/prisoner. In the law enforcement community, it occasionally becomes necessary to physically subdue an aggressive prisoner to the extent that they are hog-tied. In this position, which is only used by police in extreme cases, the patient's hands are handcuffed behind his or her back, ankle cuffs are applied, and the patient is laid face down with knees bent back so that the handcuffs and ankle cuffs can be joined together by a tie or a strap (see Figure 9-7). In this position the patient cannot strike with their arms or legs and can easily be transported to a police vehicle for transportation to a jail or similar detention facility. Unfortunately, there have been documented cases in which aggressive patients/prisoners have needed medical attention, and prehospital providers have allowed them to stay in this position face down on a stretcher. In one case in Illinois a number of years ago, a patient died in the back of an ambulance from positional asphyxia while in a hog-tied position. The police had the patient hog-tied when the ambulance arrived, and the paramedics left the patient in this position during transport. Upon arrival at the hospital, the patient was in a full arrest.

At the risk of creating a dispute with law enforcement agents, the prehospital provider must always remember that he or she is responsible for

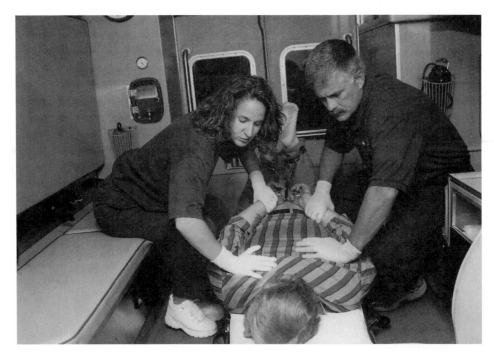

Figure 9-7 When your patient is in police custody, he or she is still your responsibility. Never allow a patient to be hog-tied and placed in your ambulance. Instead, use proper medical restraint devices and position the patient in a way that is safe for everyone.

the patient while the patient is in their custody or control, regardless of the presence or absence of incarceration. Through pre-planning and advanced discussion, prehospital providers and police officers can develop an action plan so that when an aggressive patient is placed into the back of an ambulance, the patient can be taken out of handcuffs and ankle restraints and placed in appropriate medical restraint devices. Certainly the presence and the assistance of a police officer in helping to apply the restraints is going to be welcomed and appreciated. At the same time, the prehospital provider must again remember that at this point the patient is in his or her control, and he or she will be held accountable and responsible for how the patient is managed. The techniques used to apply medical restraint devices, as opposed to handcuffs and incarcerating restraint devices, are quite different. When the person is placed on the ambulance stretcher, he or she becomes a patient and at that point medical protocol should be followed under the guidance and direction of the appropriate prehospital or other healthcare provider.

Departmental Policies

Most organizations have developed written guidelines that provide direction when assessing the need for the application of physical restraint devices. Unfortunately, while most of these directives are created with noble intention, they are often written in such a way that decisions are made long before a situation ever presents. Unfortunately, the prehospital provider who is at risk in the field becomes bound to act according to the way the policy dictates as opposed to the way the situation dictates. This is both unfortunate and unfair. Administrators of the department or the organization must evaluate how their policies are written and ensure they are written in such a way that the prehospital provider is empowered to make decisions based on the circumstances.

The prehospital provider, on the other hand, has the obligation to be familiar with and well versed in all departmental or organizational policies and procedures. It is up to the prehospital provider to follow the departmental policies and procedures at all times, as he or she will be held accountable in the event of a deviation from policy.

If the prehospital provider feels that departmental or organizational policies are unfair, unrealistic, or unenforceable, then the prehospital provider should discuss this information with management long before an incident has occurred and the prehospital provider and the organization are held accountable.

Prehospital System Standard Operating Procedures

If you work out of an established prehospital system, your system no doubt has developed systemwide standard operating procedures (SOPs). These SOPs are written by the medical director of the prehospital system to provide direction for the prehospital provider in providing medical care. The organization must assess their own SOPs against those of the prehospital system to make sure that the two are not contradictory. In the event that the two refute each other, the prehospital provider should seek out legal advice in advance. Legal advise may help determine the amount of liability exposure that the prehospital provider may face in the event that he or she fails to follow prehospital system protocols in favor of departmental protocols and vice versa.

The Reasonable Person Standard

None of us working as healthcare providers enjoy abuse at the hands of our patients. Any provider who has been cussed at, spit upon, or physically injured by a patient will tell you that maintaining control of him- or herself can be almost impossible at times. More than one healthcare provider, when dealing with an aggressive patient, has become fed up with the behavior of the patient.

For an ordinary person, the standard established by the courts is the reasonable person standard. The "reasonable person" is someone who reacts the same as any other person in the community would have acted under similar circumstances. Obviously, the reasonable person is a standard that is often difficult to judge. A split-second decision made by a healthcare professional, under highly stressful conditions, may be judged differently when a court's jury of their peers takes weeks to arrive at a conclusion.

Additionally, because the healthcare professional has specialized training and skills and is licensed/certified, they may be held at a higher standard than nonprofessional people. Providers must use a level of care that would be considered reasonable for another provider with similar skills, training, and experience. For example, if a patient becomes profane with you, would it be considered reasonable to immediately place him or her in a four-point restraint? Would this be the action that someone else with your qualifications would take? The standard of care for providers is an objective standard. If a case went to court, a jury would have to decide whether the provider made a sound decision based on his or her training and experience.

Summary

The debate over the use of restraint devices rages on. To some they are perceived as inhumane, while to others, when used properly, they are devices that serve to protect everyone, including the patient.

The healthcare professional in the twenty-first century will walk a fine line between control and abuse. Whether in the prehospital, acute-care, or long-term care setting, these professionals will be held accountable to a higher standard than ever before.

When restraints are used, they must be used in the manner for which they are intended. They cannot be used for punishment or convenience, and their use must be well documented.

If the healthcare professional is uncertain about the use of restraint devices, whether chemical or physical, a legal opinion should be obtained in the jurisdiction in which the provider operates.

CHAPTER

10

Postincident Responses

Christmas Was Just Over a Week Away

Mills Bay was a small town like so many others in the mountainous terrain of central Utah. With a population of just over 1,500, it was the kind of community where everyone in town knew everyone else. If you were a baby boomer, you'd swear you were in Mayberry. Everyone not only knew each other, but they were friendly and always willing to "pitch in" for the good of their neighbor and the community. The fire department was no different. The equipment wasn't the newest or the best, but the 25 members of the all-volunteer department worked together to make sure everything was in the best possible condition. The department wasn't just the source of firefighting and EMS for the town—it was also the focal point of the social circuit in Mills Bay. The fire hall was the main place for parties, meetings, elections, and, of course, plain, old-fashioned camaraderie.

It was another December morning, like so many others. It was sunny, yet cold, with snow on the ground. The day started off busy, at least by Mills Bay standards. There were a couple of routine wintertime calls, although two calls in one day was very rare. One was an elderly man who experienced chest pains while shoveling his sidewalk, the other a young girl who slipped on the ice and sprained her ankle. The ambulance had just returned from the hospital, and we were all sitting around the station talking about Christmas, just over a week away. Bill Wells, one of those guys you can't help but like, was talking about all the money he spent on toys for his three kids. He'd be paying off Christmas bills well into next year. He said it was well worth it though, just to see the look on their faces when they opened them. You could see the sincerity in his eyes and hear it in his voice when he talked about it. He said that's when he really appreciates being a daddy. Everyone on the department knew Bill's kids. He was so proud of them. Someone once asked him why he and his wife never took weekend trips alone, and he clearly pointed out that theirs was a family unit and would stay that way. He and his wife Sarah took the kids everywhere with them. They were so much in love with each other, their kids, and life. They were the perfect family. Everyone on the department envied their life, and I think we all appreciated our own families even more because of the way Bill and Sarah rubbed off on us.

Then the call came in that would change all of our lives forever. All the preplanning in the world never prepared us for what we were about to experience. We were dispatched to the scene of a one-car accident. The car apparently slid off the road, went through a guardrail, and started down a cliff. The car was about 10 feet down the cliff when the ambulance arrived. Thank goodness there was a huge rock that kept the vehicle from plunging to the bottom. The drop off was about 100 feet. The car had snow covering the bottom, so we couldn't see the license plate or identify the type of vehicle, but it somehow looked familiar. We grabbed a rope from the ambulance and tied one end to the piece of guardrail that seemed intact. We tied the other end to the wrecked vehicle to prevent the car from careening down the side of the cliff. The guardrail seemed stable, even though it had been broken. At the time, there was just nothing else we could use to secure the line. We could hear people yelling inside the dangling car, so we knew we had victims. We asked if anyone was hurt. There was no answer, only continuous screaming. The passengers were obviously in shock, possibly hurt, and extremely scared. We knew we had to work fast. We had to get someone into the vehicle to assess the victims. Bill, who had been an EMT for about eight years now, volunteered. An excellent mountain climber, Bill climbed every weekend and was not the least bit apprehensive. After strapping on all the protective equipment, Bill started down the cliff. He got to the car and shouted back: "Guys, help . . . it's my wife . . . it's Sarah . . . and the kids . . . please . . . help . . . Oh my God, it's my wife . . . my kids." Everyone was stunned. In a small town, you often take care of friends and family, but never had we dealt with something of this magnitude. This was Bill's family, but it was our family too. Bill married Sarah about six years ago. All of the older guys on the department attended the wedding. Sarah was an emergency department nurse at a hospital near Mills Bay. She was as much a part of "our" family as was Bill. She and Bill had three kids: Robert, age 5, Nancy, age 3, and their newest addition to the family, Melinda. Mindy was only 14 months old. All of Bill and Sarah's kids were special, but somehow Mindy had sort of been adopted as the firehouse mascot. I think she got tagged with that name at Halloween when Bill and Sarah brought her to the station dressed in a pair of scrubs with the name and logo of the department embroidered on the front. She looked absolutely adorable.

After reality set in, we realized that Bill should not be left alone to assess his own family. We didn't really have anyone else on scene who was as well trained as Bill, but the adrenaline was flowing and everyone wanted to help. We called mutual aid, but we knew it would be at least 15 to 30 minutes before anyone else arrived. We made the decision to send down Curt Byarley, a relatively new EMT. Curt was young but was probably in better physical condition than the rest of us. And he was the only other EMT on the scene besides Bill. Curt quickly donned a harness and started down the side of the cliff. Bill had not responded to us in over two minutes, although it seemed like hours. When Curt got to the car, he opened the door. He turned toward us and shouted: "It's Sarah. She's hysterical, but it looks like everyone is okay." Needless to say, we were all quite relieved. The reason Bill hadn't responded to us was because he was inside the car trying to calm Sarah, holding his kids, and telling them everything would be okay, although, according to Curt, his eyes were so filled with tears he probably couldn't tell his kids apart. Curt got in and helped Bill with Sarah. After Sarah was somewhat calmed down, Curt climbed back up and explained the situation to us. Curt thought Sarah had a strange look. He said: "Sarah was looking at Bill and me, but somehow it was like she either didn't see us, or *didn't recognize us. The windshield is spiderwebbed, so she may have a pretty significant head injury." We decided that Curt would go back down, and we would send down a stokes basket to remove Sarah and the kids, one-by-one.*

As Curt got back to the car, he slipped and slid into the open door. The car became a little unstable, but since it was secured to the guardrail, it didn't move much. Bill and Curt both worked feverishly to get Mindy out first. Since Mindy was only a baby and was crying at the top of her lungs, they thought it would be best if they took her out first. It might also help to calm Sarah and the other kids more. Bill and Curt got little Mindy strapped into the stretcher and were just about to bring her out when it happened. By this time, the snow on the back of the car was melted enough that we could see inside. We witnessed Sarah becoming violent, shouting and striking at Bill and Curt. She kept saying: "Don't take my baby, you bastards. Don't take my baby . . ."

Things are kind of a blur to this day, but somehow, probably from all the commotion inside the car, the guardrail failed, and their car started to roll down the side of the cliff. We tried to grab on, but by the time we noticed the guardrail failing, it was too late to stop it. George Moor, who was set to retire next month after 30 years with the department, jumped on the rope. We guess now he thought he could stop it somehow—maybe it was just an instinctive reaction. We're not sure what he was thinking. When the guardrail snapped, it struck George in the head, killing him instantly. The coroner said his neck snapped so quickly he didn't feel a thing. Free from its restraints, the car began rolling down the side of the hill. We heard their screams and watched in terror as the car fell to the ground, 100 feet below. It took less than a few seconds, but it seemed like an eternity. It was as if everything was moving in slow motion. The car landed on its top and burst into flames. Then there was nothing but silence. We could see the flames. We could see the wheels still spinning on the car, but we knew by the silence that they were all gone. By the time we got to them, it was too late. They were all dead. Bill, Sarah, Robert, Nancy, little Mindy, Curt, and George. Two families were wiped out—theirs, and ours.

My mind is now like a videocassette player. The tape just plays over and over and over in my head. I can't seem to shake it—and it's been four years since the accident. It won't go away. . . .

Introduction

Okay! You've done everything correctly. You've implemented the PREVENT®
plan for violence, including personal vulnerability, equipment, vehicle, and
self-assessments. You know how to recognize potential violence. You've
learned the aggression continuum and proper response techniques. You've
implemented the team intervention concept. You've even learned and prac-
ticed defensive techniques, including proper restraint methods. Therefore,
you can't possibly become a victim of violence, can you?

Once again, think about the profession you've chosen. Although it is one you should be very proud of, it is also one in which violence is growing, no matter how small or how large your department may be. Violence comes in all shapes and sizes. It has no biases. Violence victimizes people of all religions, ethnicities, moral principles, and economic status. You might tell yourself, "I've seen it all. Nothing can possibly affect me. I've breathed air into the lungs of a dying child, I've pulled mangled bodies out of cars. I've confronted death numerous times in my career, and have never been adversely affected. How could violence possibly affect me?" If you still think you can't become a victim of violence, you better think again.

Posttraumatic Stress Disorder

People grieve in different ways. Some are quiet and show little emotion. Some are very emotional, shouting and yelling, sometimes kicking, throwing, and even punching things. Some faint. Still others burst out in tears. Yet, in some cases, feelings of loss may not show up until several weeks or months after a tragic event. This is called posttraumatic stress disorder (PTSD).

According to the National Institute of Mental Health, PTSD is a debilitating condition that follows a terrifying event. People with PTSD often have persistent frightening thoughts and memories of their ordeal and feel emotionally numb, especially when it involves people to whom they were once close. War veterans first brought PTSD, once referred to as shell shock or battle fatigue, to public attention, but it can result from any number of traumatic incidents. These include kidnapping; serious accidents such as car or train wrecks; natural disasters such as floods, tornadoes, or earthquakes; and violent attacks such as a mugging, sexual assault, torture, or being held captive. The event that triggers it may be something that threatened the person's life or the life of someone close to him or her. Or it could be something witnessed, such as the mass death and destruction that often follows a plane crash.

Whatever the source of the problem, some people with PTSD repeatedly relive the trauma in the form of nightmares and disturbing recollections during the day. They may also experience sleep problems, depression, feelings of detachment or numbness, or being easily startled. They may lose interest in things they used to enjoy and have trouble feeling affectionate. They may feel irritable, more aggressive than before, or even violent. Seeing things that remind them of the incident may be very distressing, and can lead them to avoid certain places or situations that bring back those memories. Anniversaries of the event are often very difficult.

PTSD can occur at any age, including childhood. Depression, substance abuse, or anxiety can accompany the disorder. Symptoms may be mild or severe; people may become easily irritated or have violent outbursts. In severe cases they may have trouble working or socializing. In general, the symptoms seem to be worse if it is a person that committed the act, such as in a sexual assault, as opposed to one cause by a natural disaster.

Ordinary events can serve as reminders of the trauma and trigger flashbacks or intrusive images. A flashback may make the person lose touch with reality and reenact the event for a period of seconds or hours or, very rarely, days. A person having a flashback, which can come in the form of images, sounds, smells, or feelings, usually believes that the traumatic event is happening all over again.

Not every traumatized person gets full-blown PTSD, or even experiences PTSD at all. PTSD is diagnosed only if the symptoms last more than a month. In those who do have PTSD, symptoms usually begin within three months of the trauma, and the course of the illness varies. Some people recover within six months; others have symptoms that last much longer. In some cases, the condition may be chronic. Occasionally, the illness doesn't show up until years after the traumatic event.

Antidepressants and anxiety-reducing medications can ease the symptoms of depression and sleep problems, and psychotherapy, including cognitive–behavioral therapy, is an integral part of treatment. Being exposed to a reminder of the trauma as part of therapy, such as returning to the scene of a sexual assault, sometimes helps. And support from family and friends can help speed recovery.

The American Counseling Association (ACA) is the largest private, nonprofit organization for professional counselors in the world. Founded in 1952, their services include leadership training, continuing education, and advocacy services. The ACA offers the following 10 signs and symptoms of PTSD. Recognizing these symptoms is the first step toward recovery:

1. Reexperiencing the event through vivid memories or flashbacks
2. Feeling emotionally numb
3. Feeling overwhelmed by what would normally be considered everyday situations and diminished interest in performing normal tasks or pursuing usual interests
4. Crying uncontrollably
5. Isolating oneself from family and friends and avoiding social situations
6. Relying increasingly on alcohol or drugs to get through the day
7. Feeling extremely moody, irritable, angry, suspicious, or frightened
8. Having difficulty falling or staying asleep, sleeping too much, and experiencing nightmares
9. Feeling guilty about surviving the event or being unable to solve the problem, change the event, or prevent the disaster
10. Feeling fears and sense of doom about the future

Once the symptoms are identified and the need for treatment recognized, the question remains, what can be done to help the troubled provider? Healthcare professionals can manage the stress brought on by everyday events in the following ways. First and foremost, don't wait for an event or an accumulation of events to occur before you decide to reduce work-related stress. Having a profound awareness of the problem and educating yourself as much as possible on coping skills will go a long way to reducing stress. In addition, get plenty of rest and relaxation and start an exercise program. Many providers also get caught up in their work and tend to carry the burden of the world on their shoulders. Although there never seems to be enough time in the day, it is wise to have a life outside your work. Spend more time with your family, go to or participate in your kids' school activities or sporting events, watch a sitcom, read a good book (preferably not work-related), volunteer your time for a needy cause or church function, or engage in some other activity enjoyable and rewarding to you. No matter what activity you choose, avoid the use of drugs and alcohol. Resorting to drugs and alcohol may seemingly ease the pain, but they are likely to intensify your ill feelings or cloud your judgment while under their influence.

Critical Incident Stress Debriefings

Much is written about critical incident stress debriefings (CISDs). As explained by Mitchell and Everly (1995), CISD is the process of providing intervention and education following an event that has had a stressful impact sufficient enough to overwhelm the usually effective coping skills of either an individual or a group.

Critical incident stress debriefing:
- is not therapy or a substitute for therapy.
- should be applied only by those who have been specifically trained in its uses.
- is a group process, group meeting, or discussion designed to reduce stress and enhance recovery from stress. It is based on principles of crisis intervention and education.
- may not solve all the problems presented during the brief time-frame available.
- may indicate that sometimes it will be necessary to refer individuals for therapy treatment after a debriefing.
- may accelerate the rate of normal recovery, in normal people, who are having normal reactions to abnormal events.

There is significant argument over the use of CISDs. Some say CISDs help prevent the onset of PTSD. Others say CISDs are not helpful and may even increase the amount of stress from a critical incident. One way to handle PTSD is to offer a variety of options.

Let employees choose which option they want. For some employees, CISDs may be very useful, while others may have their own coping mechanisms already in place. These may include family, friends, clergy, or others with whom they are comfortable communicating. Many organizations enlist the services of employee assistance programs, crisis intervention teams, peer groups, or other agencies specializing in posttraumatic intervention. A brief explanation of these options follows.

Employee Assistance Programs

Employee Assistance Programs (EAPs) normally provide professional counseling services for employees and their families who are experiencing personal problems that may be affecting job performance. The programs offer assessment, referral, short-term counseling, and follow-up for employees and families confronted with the following:

- Drug/alcohol-related problems
- Family problems
- Economic problems
- Stress
- Mental illness

Some even offer expert advice on eating a balanced diet, weight loss, and smoking cessation.

Crisis Intervention Teams

Crisis intervention teams vary from EAPs in that they normally respond to a sudden, catastrophic event. Crisis intervention teams may be a part of an existing EAP, but currently they rarely are used to help employees with cumulative exposure to traumatic events. As cumulative trauma becomes more widely recognized, we are starting to see a shift from crisis intervention to crisis management. Cumulative trauma is the incessant exposure to death, traumatic events, and violence, in addition to the everyday stresses most of us face.

Peer Groups

Peer groups are normally made up of others in the same line of work, often within the same department, who are better able to understand the specific circumstances of a traumatic event. Like crisis intervention teams, they normally focus on a specific event. Many are led by professional counselors with expertise in PTSD.

Other Agencies

There are numerous agencies available to assist you and your department with postincident interventions. The government funds many of them, and their services are often free. Even more agencies are available on a fee-for-service basis. You can find information on both at your local library, on the Internet, or from local police, fire, prehospital, and participating healthcare facilities.

No matter what type of services you choose for yourself or for your employees, the objectives should be to accomplish the following:

- Confidential counseling on matters affecting the physical and emotional well-being of employees and their families. (These may or may not be job-related matters.)
- Improved work performance by relieving the day-to-day stress employees face.
- Retention of valuable employees.
- Enhancement of the work environment.
- Enhancement of the home environment.

Keep in mind that none of the options discussed earlier are fully inclusive nor should they take the place of professional counseling. If you, your family, or any other person suffers from stress, it would be wise to seek professional assistance. Your primary physician will likely have a list of referrals. If not, many healthcare facilities can provide you with the names of qualified professionals.

Summary

You may never be as prepared for traumatic incidents as you think you are. Nevertheless, understand that violence is here to stay, and that no matter how hard-hearted you think you are, violence can affect you. By implementing programs of awareness and prevention, and seeking assistance when symptoms occur, you, your family, and co-workers will be less likely to have long-term effects from exposure to traumatic events.

Reference

Mitchell, J.T., and Everly, G.S. (1995). *Critical Incident Stress Debriefing: An Operations Manual for the Prevention of Trauma Among Emergency Service and Disaster Workers.* (2nd ed.). Baltimore, MD: Chevron.

Epilogue

Aggressive behavior is not going to be removed from our society. For whatever reasons, all of us who care for the physical and emotional needs of others will from time to time be faced with an individual who presents a threat to us. Our safety, and perhaps our survival, will depend on how we respond.

The material contained in this text evolved from a continuing education class developed to help a prehospital agency that was experiencing high injury rates at the hands of aggressive patients. Soon after, word of the program spread, and we were inundated with requests for this training. It became obvious to us that after years of training hospital professionals, it was time to pay attention to the prehospital providers as well.

We have both worked our entire careers in emergency services and healthcare safety management. From basic emergency medical technicians school all the way through paramedic school, aggression management was mentioned *but never taught*. At the time, mental health facilities were closing, and the focus was shifting to outpatient treatment. Prehospital providers were frequently injured at the hands of aggressive patients, but little was done to help prepare them to deal with these special patients.

In this text, we have tried to focus on the three main areas of healthcare that deal with aggressive behaviors: prehospital, acute care, and long-term care. Throughout we use examples based on actual case studies that the authors have either been involved in or made aware of. Even though the examples and text may address or reference one group of professionals, the techniques discussed can be applied universally.

Finally, for your own safety, we want to again point out that the defensive tactics introduced in this text are just that—an introduction. Reading the text and "trying the techniques" does not constitute developing proficiency. We encourage the use of these techniques, but only after you have been trained under the guidance of a qualified instructor.

Steve Wilder, CHSP, EMT-P
Chris Sorensen, CHPA

Sorensen, Wilder & Associates
596 N. Van Buren Avenue
Bradley, Illinois 60915
Voice: 800-568-2931
Fax: 815-933-1464
e-mail: swainc@keynet.net
www.swa4safety.com

Index

F

Face down position, 114
Facial muscles, twitching of, 85
Five-point restraint, 134
Fixed staring, 85
Flashback, 143
Four-point restraint, 133–34
Front chokehold, techniques to avoid, 102–3
Front hair grab, 96–97
   takedown from, 120
Front windmill technique, 103

G

Gang violence in hospital, 33–34
Geographic locating devices, 42
Grabs
   clothing, 98–100
      takedown from, 121
   front hair, 96–97
      takedown from, 120
   one-hand wrist, 93–94
      takedown from, 119–20
   rear hair, 97–98
      takedown from, 120–21
   of stethoscopes, 101
   two-hand wrist, 95
      takedown from, 120

H

Hair grab
   front, 96–97
      takedown from, 120
   rear, 97–98
      takedown from, 120–21
Haldol, 127
Handshake hold, 95
Hazard prevention and controls,
   development of, in OSHA Workplace
   Violence Standard, 9–13
Headlock, 107–9
Healthcare professionals, use of force by, 112–13
High kick block
   from defensive stance, 116
   from interview stance, 116
Holds, escapes from, 88–110
Hospital-affiliated skilled nursing facilities,
   restraint use in, 126
Hospitals
   restraint use in, 126
   violence in, 24–35
      bomb threats and civil unrest, 34–35
      community, 30–31
      domestic, 31–33
      employee against employee, 30
      gang, 33–34
      patient against employee, 26–27
      patient against patient, 28–29
      visitor against employee, 28
      visitor against patient, 29–30

I

Incident reports, 14–15
Individual versus team, 65
Initial interview stance, 114
Injury reports, assessing, in preventing violence, 41
Innocent bystander protection, 62
Instructions, keeping minimal, 77
Instrument pouches, 12
Interview stance
   high kick block from, 116
   low kick block from, 115
   middle kick block from, 116
Inverted V technique, 102

J

Jacket restraint, 128

K

Kicks, blocking, 115–16

L

Law enforcement officers, presence of, in hospital, 34
Legal considerations, restraints and, 126–27
Librium, 127
Long-term care, restraint use in, 126–27
Low kick block
   from defensive stance, 116
   from interview stance, 115

M

Management commitment and employee involvement in OSHA Workplace Violence Standard, 8–9
Medical care, providing quality, 72
Medical reports, 14
Mental health units, violence in, 27
Middle kick block from interview stance, 116
Mitten restraint, 130
Muscle groups, tightening of small and large, 84–85

N

Nonthreatening behavior, 53, 72–73
Nonverbal clues of impending physical violence, 84–85
Nursing homes, restraint use in, 126

O

Occupational Safety and Health Administration (OSHA)
   on incidents of domestic violence, 5–6
   workplace violence prevention guidelines, 30